OPPRESSION

OPPRESSION

A Social Determinant of Health

Edited by

Elizabeth A. McGibbon

Fernwood Publishing • Halifax & Winnipeg

Cover design: John van der Woude
Cover photo copyright © Riley Smith Photography
Printed and bound in Canada by Hignell Book Printing

Published in Canada by Fernwood Publishing
32 Oceanvista Lane, Black Point, Nova Scotia, B0J 1B0
and 748 Broadway Avenue, Winnipeg, Manitoba, R3G 0X3
www.fernwoodpublishing.ca

Fernwood Publishing Company Limited gratefully acknowledges the financial support of
the Government of Canada through the Canada Book Fund and the Canada Council for the Arts,
the Nova Scotia Department of Communities, Culture and Heritage, the Manitoba Department of
Culture, Heritage and Tourism under the Manitoba Publishers Marketing Assistance Program and
the Province of Manitoba, through the Book Publishing Tax Credit, for our publishing program.

 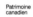

Library and Archives Canada Cataloguing in Publication

McGibbon, Elizabeth Anne, 1955-
Oppression: a social determinant of health / Elizabeth A. McGibbon.

Includes bibliographical references.
ISBN 978-1-55266-454-4 (bound).--ISBN 978-1-55266-445-2 (pbk.)

1. Health--Social aspects. 2. Health--Political aspects. 3. Medical economics.
4. Oppression (Psychology)--Health aspects. I. Title.

RA418.M26 2012   306.4'61   C2011-908390-6

Contents

Contributors... 9

Preface and Acknowledgements 14

Part 1: Politicizing Health

1   Introduction to Oppression and the Social Determinants of Health
    Elizabeth McGibbon 16

    The Moral Imperative of a Critical Perspective 18
    Overview of the Book 22
    Defining Oppression 24
    An Example: The Oppression of Women 25
    The Cycle of Oppression 27

2. People under Threat: Health Outcomes and Oppression
    Elizabeth A. McGibbon 32

    Reframing "Vulnerable People" as "People under Threat" 33
    How Oppression Is Inscribed on Body and Mind 33
    Synergies of Oppression: A Framework for Tackling SDH Inequities 40
    Anchoring Change in the Structural Determinants of Health 44

3. Critical Perspectives on the Social Determinants of Health
    Dennis Raphael 45

    Defining the Social Determinants of Health 47
    Differing SDH Discourses 49
    Conclusion 59

Part 2: How Oppression Operates to Produce Health Inequities

4. Fragmented Performances:Ageism and the Health of Older Women
    Raewyn Bassett 62

    The Health of Women Aged Sixty-Five and Over 63
    Discourses about Aging 66
    Ageism 68
    Fragmented Performances 71

5. Race and Racism as Determinants of Health
    Josephine B. Etowa & Elizabeth A. McGibbon........................... 73
    Inscribing Racism on Body and Mind.. 74
    How Do Race and Racism Determine Health? 77
    Racism and Health: A Social Determinants Perspective......................... 79
    Conclusions 87

6. Oppression and the Health of Indigenous Peoples
    Marie Battiste & James [Sa'ke'j] Youngblood Henderson........................... 89
    The Impact of Psychosocial Stress... 91
    Racialization 92
    Neocolonization and Eurocentric Analytical Systems......................... 95
    Conclusion... 96

7. Social Exclusion as a Determinant of Health
    Grace-Edward Galabuzi.. 97
    Social Determinants of Health and Social Exclusion......................... 98
    Defining Social Exclusion... 99
    Dimensions of Exclusion 100
    Conclusion... 112

8. Oppression and Im/migrant Health in Canada
    Denise Spitzer 113
    Im/migrating to Canada 115
    Im/migrant Lives in Canada 116
    Im/migrant Health and Well-Being in Canada 118
    Oppression, Health and the Embodiment of Inequality 120
    Resisting Oppression.. 121
    Conclusion... 122
    Notes... 122

9. Oppression and Mental Health: Pathologizing the Outcomes of Injustice
    Elizabeth A. McGibbon 123
    Mental Health Outcomes of
    Oppression-Related Spiritual and Psychological Stress......................... 124
    Pathologizing the Mental Health Consequences of Oppression 131
    Intergenerational Trauma Transmission and Oppressed Peoples......................... 134
    Conclusions 137

10. Oppression, Health and Public Policy in Canada
    Toba Bryant 138
    What Is Public Policy?.. 139
    Social Inequalities and the Welfare State............................... 145
    Income Transfers and Benefits In-Kind................................. 147
    Conclusion... 148

11. A Rights-Based Approach to Primary Health Care: Increasing Accountability for Health Inequities within Health Systems Strengthening
Charmaine McPherson 150

Health Equity, Primary Health Care and a Human Rights-Based Approach..... 151
Linkages among Health, Health Equity and Human Rights................................. 154
A Rights-Based Approach to Furthering Health Equity 155
Embedding a Rights-Based Approach in Primary Health Care............................ 160
Major Issues Hindering an RBA in Primary Health Care Renewal 161
A Way Forward on Health Inequities and Primary Health Care Renewal 165

12. Oppression and the Political Economy of Health Inequities
Elizabeth A. McGibbon and Lars K. Hallstrom 167

Epidemiological Perspectives on Population Health 168
Political Economy and a Materialist Perspective on Health 169
Health and Public Policy from a Structural Perspective 171
Policy Implications for Reducing Health Inequities 182
Health Policy by Design.. 184
Conclusions 185

13. Health as Human Right: Challenges and Supports for Accountability
Elizabeth A. McGibbon & Maureen Shebib 186

Health as a Human Right: Core Concepts 187
Canadian Human Rights Instruments and the Right to Health............................ 189
International Human Rights Law 200
Conclusions 203

Select Bibliography 204

To my daughters,
Emily Eugenie Gardner and Sophie Margaret Gardner,
ever inspirations that a just and compassionate society
is at hand.

Contributors

Raewyn Bassett, PhD, is a sociologist in the Faculty of Health Professions at Dalhousie University, Halifax, Nova Scotia. Her research interests include social inequalities, social identities, memory and aging. A qualitative researcher, Raewyn also has a substantive interest in the use of qualitative software programs in the development of qualitative research methodologies and methods.

Marie Battiste, a Mi'kmaw educator from Potlo'tek First Nation, is full professor in the College of Education and Coordinator of the Indian and Northern Education Program within Educational Foundations at the University of Saskatchewan. She is acting director of the Humanities Research Unit at the University of Saskatchewan. Her historical research of Mi'kmaw literacy and education as a graduate student at Harvard University and later at Stanford University, where she received her doctorate degree in curriculum and teacher education, provided the foundation for her later writings on cognitive imperialism, linguistic and cultural integrity and decolonization of Aboriginal education. A recipient of two honorary degrees from St. Mary's University and from her alma mater, University of Maine at Farmington, she has worked actively with First Nations schools and communities as an administrator, teacher, consultant and curriculum developer, advancing Aboriginal epistemology, languages, pedagogy and research. Her research interests are in initiating institutional change in the decolonization of education, language and social justice policy and power, and education approaches that recognize and affirm the political and cultural diversity of Canada and the ethical protection of Indigenous knowledge.

Toba Bryant is an assistant professor of health studies at the University of Toronto Scarborough. Dr. Bryant received an honours bachelor's degree in political science, followed by an MSW and PhD in social work with a specialization in public policy. She has published extensively on health and social policy change, social and health inequalities, and women's health issues. She is the sole author of *An Introduction to Health Policy.* She is also a co-editor of *Staying Alive: Critical Perspectives on Health, Illness, and Health Care,* and a contributor to *Social Determinants of Health: Canadian Perspectives.* She was co-editor of two special journal issues: "Social Inequalities and Health" in *Humanity & Society* and "Population Health in the Twenty-first Century" in *Social Alternatives.*

Josephine B. Etowa is an associate professor at the University of Ottawa's Faculty of Health Sciences, School of Nursing. Dr Etowa completed her BSc. N and MN degrees from Dalhousie University and her PhD in nursing at the University of Calgary. She completed a Canadian Health Services Research Foundation (CHSRF) post-doctoral fellowship focusing on diversity within Canadian nursing at the University of Toronto and the University of Ottawa. Her research program, which is grounded in over twenty-three years of clinical practice, is in the area of inequity in health and health care as well as maternal-newborn health. Her research projects have been funded by international, national, provincial and local agencies, and these projects are guided by the tenets of qualitative research and participatory action research (PAR).

Grace-Edward Galabuzi is an associate professor in the Department of Politics and Public Administration at Ryerson University. He is also a research associate at the Centre for Social Justice in Toronto. In addition to a PhD (political science) from York University, he also holds a BA in economics from the University of Winnipeg, a BA (Honours) in political science from York University and an MA in political science from York University. His current teaching areas include equity and human rights and third world politics. He has previously taught at York University (international relations) and George Brown College (anti-racism, multiculturalism and local politics). His research interests include globalization from below — local community responses to global economic restructuring in the global North and South; the racialization of the Canadian labour market; and social exclusion and the social economic status of racialized groups in Canada.

Lars K. Hallstrom is the director of the Alberta Centre for Sustainable Rural Communities, a new and joint initiative of the Augustana Faculty of the University of Alberta in Camrose and the Faculty of Agriculture, Life and Environmental Sciences at the main campus in Edmonton. A specialist in comparative environmental policy and politics, Dr. Hallstrom's research has focused on the intersection of science and public participation in the public-policy process. He has published widely on a number of topics, including the politics and enlargement of the European Union, environmental and democratic theory, forest resources management and genetically modified foods, and has received grants from funders such as SSHRC, CIHR, PHAC and the NSHRF. In 2006, Dr. Hallstrom led the team that was awarded federal funding to establish the National Collaborating Centre for Determinants of Health in Nova Scotia, and he served as its acting director until returning to full-time research in 2007.

James [Sa'ke'j] Youngblood Henderson was born to the Bear Clan of the Chickasaw Nation and Cheyenne Tribe in Oklahoma in 1944 and is married to Marie Battiste, a Mi'kmaw educator. They have three children. In 1974, he received a juris doctorate in law from Harvard Law School and became a law professor who created litigation strategies to restore Aboriginal culture, institutions and rights. He co-authored the book *The Road, Indian Tribes and Political Liberty* and has written many law review articles on Indian issues. During the constitutional process (1978–1993) in Canada, he served as a constitutional advisor for the Mikmaw nation and the NIB-Assembly of First Nations. He has continued to develop in the areas of Aboriginal and treaty rights and treaty federalism in constitutional law. His latest books are *Aboriginal Tenure in the Constitution of Canada* (2000) and *Protecting Indigenous Knowledge and Heritage* (2000). He is working on *Treaty rights in the Constitution of Canada* (2002). He is a noted international human rights lawyer and an authority on protecting Indigenous heritage, knowledge and culture. He was one of the drafters and expert advisors of the principles and guidelines for the protection of Indigenous heritage in the U.N. Human Rights fora.

Elizabeth A. McGibbon, RN, PhD, is an associate professor at St. Francis Xavier University, Antigonish, Nova Scotia. Elizabeth lives with her husband, Patrick Gardner, and their daughters, Emily Eugenie and Sophie Margaret. Her CIHR, CHSRF and NDHRF funded studies focus on critical social science applications to health issues: public-policy and health disparities related to the social determinants of health; tackling health disparities through public health systems strengthening; human rights and health; access to health services; gender, racism and health; and geography and health. Her knowledge of health inequity and its impact on health outcomes of racialized and marginalized peoples is based in over twenty years of mental health clinical practice and working for change in large institutions and in the community. She was one of three lead authors of the successful Public Health Agency of Canada's National Collaborating Centre for the Social Determinants of Health. She has published nationally recognized critical works in the sociology of health and illness, including *Anti-racist Health Care Practice* (co-authored with Josephine B. Etowa).

Charmaine McPherson is an associate professor in the School of Nursing at St. Francis Xavier University, completed a PhD at McMaster University in Hamilton, Ontario, and an MSc with a clinical nurse specialty in psychiatry at Boston College, Massachusetts. She is a primary health care and public-policy expert specializing in interorganizational and cross-sectoral network partnerships to advance population health and health equity within a social justice frame. Dr. McPherson brings a unique blend of twenty-two years of administrative and clinical practice in community mental health, NGO community-based residential care and regional interorganizational child health networks to her applied health research program. She has contributed to many rural social justice and health efforts through local, national and international organizations and partnerships. She has conducted more than a hundred invited and peer-reviewed presentations. She also advances innovative organizational planning and development through her private practice, ENS Consulting.

Dennis Raphael, PhD, is a professor of health policy and management at York University in Toronto. The most recent of his over 150 scientific publications have focused on the health effects of income inequality and poverty, the quality of life of communities and individuals, and the impact of government decisions on Canadians' health and well-being. Dr. Raphael is editor of *Social Determinants of Health: Canadian Perspectives* (now in second edition), co-editor of *Staying Alive: Critical Perspectives on Health, Illness, and Health Care* (now in second edition) and author of *Poverty and Policy in Canada: Implications for Health and Quality of Life*, all published by Canadian Scholars' Press. He is also the editor of *Health Promotion and Quality of Life in Canada: Essential Readings* and the author of *About Canada: Health and Illness.*

Maureen Shebib has her LLB and LLM from Dalhousie University Law School. Her specialty areas are human rights, employment equity and administrative law. She has been the human rights and equity officer at St. Francis Xavier and at Mount Saint Vincent Universities. She was in-house legal counsel to the NS Human Rights Commission for six years and a Canadian human rights (act) tribunal adjudicator for three years. She co-taught at Dalhousie University Law School and Mount Saint Vincent in the areas of poverty and family law. She taught an online course through Dalhousie University Continuing Education Department. Ms. Shebib currently works with Investigation and Complaint Services, Nova Scotia Office of the Ombudsman. She also continues a private practice as an investigator, trainer and mediator.

Denise Spitzer, PhD, is the Canada research chair in gender, migration and health, an associate professor with the Institute of Women's Studies and a principal scientist in the Institute of Population Health. In addition to undergraduate studies in biology, Chinese and music, she holds graduate degrees in anthropology. Dr. Spitzer is interested in how global processes — intersecting with gender, ethnicity, migration status and other social identifiers — are implicated in health and well-being. With the support of graduate students, academic investigators and community partners, Dr. Spitzer's current research focuses on immigrant and refugee women and engages with critical perspectives of the body; transnationalism and identity; the impact of policy on health; agency and social support; community-based research; and gender and diversity-based analysis.

Preface and Acknowledgements

The evidence and discussions in this book underscore the urgent need to reframe health inequities explicitly within the context of systemic oppression. Although there is increasing discussion in Canada about differences in health outcomes and how they may be related to social inequalities, there is a continued reluctance and resistance to identifying the "causes of the causes" of differentials in health outcomes across race, social class, gender, sexual orientation and age — racism, classism, sexism and misogyny, heterosexism and homophobic hatred, and ageism — among others. We have barely begun to talk about the intersections of these oppressions and the ways that their powerful synergy impacts health and well-being. This book contributes to the small but growing field of critical health studies in Canada, where the focus is on political ideologies and resultant public policy, which persistently supports oppressive social and material conditions.

My compass for this book rests in my years of clinical work on the pointy edges of material and social deprivation — community health centres, centres for homeless young people and inpatient/outpatient mental health clinics and institutions. In order to make meaning of what I witnessed, early on I discovered that the sheer enormity of unfairness and relentless everyday injustices must surely have a source, a catalyst, an engine. This is where change must happen. The more we (civil society, public policymakers, practitioners in the health and human services, researchers) know about the details of how oppression operates, the more we are able to tackle it. The writings in this book bring the reader into the realm of these details, with statistical and qualitative evidence, careful attention to theoretical notions that are important in understanding the mechanisms of oppression and a clear solution-based focus.

I would like to acknowledge the ongoing support and encouragement of Errol Sharpe and the copyediting and production team at Fernwood: Brenda Conroy, Beverley Rach, John van der Woude and Debbie Mathers. I also wish to thank the astute editorial support of Olga Gladkikh, whose life work is also in the area of social justice and community development. Last but certainly not least, I thank my cadre of critical readers, whose expertise in various areas was much appreciated in the editing of the chapters that I had a hand in: Emily Gardner, Sophie Gardner, Patrick Gardner, Wendy Panagopolous and Patty Smith. I have the privilege of drawing on their collective broad base of wisdom — not only in relation to this book.

Part 1

Politicizing Health

Overview of Oppression as a Social Determinant of Health

1

Introduction to Oppression and the Social Determinants of Health

Elizabeth McGibbon

Economic and racial inequality are not abstract concepts, [they] hospitalize and kill even more people than cigarettes. The wages and benefits we're paid, the neighborhoods we live in, the schools we attend, our access to resources and even our tax policies are health issues every bit as critical as diet, smoking, and exercise. The unequal distribution of these social conditions, and their health consequences, are not natural or inevitable. They are the result of choices that we as a community, as states, and as a nation have made, and can make differently. Other nations already have, and they live longer, healthier lives as a result. (Larry Adelman, executive producer, *Unnatural Causes*, 2008)

The mental, physical and spiritual suffering caused by oppression is not inevitable. However, its perpetuation is well entrenched in health and public policy and in the mechanisms for distribution of the necessities of life, including the health and legal systems, which purport to alleviate this suffering. These processes are core causes of increasing health inequities in Canada and globally. Yes, being overweight and smoking can cause heart disease. But why is the incidence of smoking and obesity so tethered to social class? Yes, lack of formal education results in significantly lower life chances. But why is lack of educational achievement so racialized? The authors of this book tackle these kinds of questions with a frank and critical perspective to expose the "causes of the causes" of health inequities as well as some of the beneficiaries of persistent systemic oppression. The overall goal of the book is to support, enhance, and provoke action to interrogate oppression and to continue to take action to halt its progress. It can be done, and it is being done.

This introductory chapter describes some important foundations of the book. I stress the moral imperative of a critical perspective because this approach keeps the analytical gaze focused on the systemic causes of ill health. I define oppression and include a detailed account of the cycle of oppression. The morally reprehensible treatment of Indigenous peoples in Canada illustrates how this cycle operates to reinforce oppression. The book uses the

Table 1.1: The Social Determinants of Health

Employment and working conditions, i.e., meaningful employment, work safety, dependable and consistent work. Women with disabilities are twice as likely to be unemployed (Statistics Canada, 2005a). Immigrant women face numerous stressors, such as finding employment and establishing income, which can have a serious health impact (Meadows, Thurston, & Melton, 2001).

Income and its equitable distribution, i.e., adequate annual income and a family's capacity to meet basic needs. Overall income of most Canadian families has steadily decreased since 1986 (Curry-Stevens, 2001). One out of four First Nations children live in poverty (Campaign 2000, 2010).

Food security, i.e., a family's capacity to consistently provide sufficient, nutritious and fresh foods. Food bank use doubled between 1989 and 2004. Forty-one percent of food bank users are children under eighteen (Toronto Charter, 2003). Child hunger is an extreme example of family food insecurity (McIntyre, 2004). People who experience food insecurity are significantly more likely to have Type II diabetes (Seligman, Bindman, Vittinghoff et al. 2007).

Housing, i.e., consistent, stable, safe shelter and green space for play. As more Canadians spend more income on shelter, housing security is threatened. Canada's renter households have average incomes that are half that of home owners (Shapcott & Hulchanski, 2004). Damp housing further exacerbates health problems such as childhood asthma (Bryant, Chisholm, & Crowe, 2002).

Early childhood development, education and care, i.e., nurturing and abuse free environments, access to appropriate child-care supports and early childhood education. Early childhood development is threatened due to continuing levels of family poverty (Raphael, 2004). Public investment does not adequately support early childhood education opportunities (McPherson, Popp, & Lindstrom, 2006).

Education, i.e., opportunity for post-secondary education. Average yearly university tuition has tripled since 1991 (Statistics Canada, 2007). Health literacy is strongly related to level of formal education, health outcomes and access to care. Except for Nova Scotia, Atlantic provinces have lower literacy rates than the national average (Murray, Rudd, Kirsch, et al. 2007).

Table 1.1: The Social Determinants of Health

Health services, i.e., culturally safe access to primary health care, specialist and multi-disciplinary services. Rural people have less access to health services and have poorer health than urban people. Women living in the most rural areas are most likely to report fair/poor health (CIHI, 2006). Racism in health care is an important barrier in access to health services (Etowa, Weins, Bernard et al., 2007).

Social inclusion, i.e., access to social supports and community participation. Groups experiencing social exclusion tend to sustain higher health risks and lower health status. These groups include Indigenous people, immigrants, refugees, persons of colour, persons with disabilities, lone parents, children, youth in disadvantaged circumstances, women, the elderly, unpaid caregivers, gays, lesbians, bisexuals, transgendered people (Galabuzi, 2006). Note that many of these groups are also included in "identity" below.

Social safety nets, i.e., access to income supplements and publicly funded home-care support. For example, the Maritime provinces have the lowest per-person spending on home care in Canada (Coyte & McKeever, 2001). Home care has been left out of the national policy agenda, which has grave consequences for the health of many vulnerable populations, including elders, and chronically ill children (Shamian, 2007).

Identity, i.e., gender, race, ethnicity, culture, age, social class, (dis)ability, sexual orientation, and age, to name a few, all determine health care access and health outcomes. Gender and race have recently been added to earlier definitions of this SDH. These definitions have been expanded to include the broader notion of identity as an SDH (McGibbon, Etowa, & McPherson, 2008a).

Toronto Charter's social determinants of health (SDH) (Raphael 2009a), as revised by Mikkonen and Raphael (2010), with the addition of identity as an SDH (McGibbon and Etowa 2009). Table 1.1 describes these SDH, with an emphasis on Canadian evidence.

The Moral Imperative of a Critical Perspective

Although there is a substantial literature about power and oppression, analysis of the explicit links between social structures and the health of citizens has only recently garnered sustained national and international attention. This new field of critical health studies aims to interrogate taken-for-granted ideas about human health and the genesis of psychological and physical wellness and illness. Emphasis on the social determinants of health focuses the gaze on the historical, political, social and economic antecedents of ill health. Unfortunately, policymakers and others have progressed at a snail's pace since eighteenth-century physician Rudolf Virchow's famous claim: "All diseases have two causes — one pathological and the other political."

Resistance to critical perspectives on health is deeply embedded in societal systems. The reasons for this resistance are complex and interrelated. Biomedical dominance has played, and continues to play, a pivotal role in keeping the analytic focus in the area of acute (i.e., hospital-based) care and at the level of the individual body. In modern Western societies, despite rhetoric about prevention, hospital-based care consumes most health care money, and hospitals are organized around individual body systems and parts: the heart unit (cardiology), the bones unit (orthopedics), the urinary tract unit (urology) and so on. This model is so entrenched that it is difficult to envision the geography of redesigned intersectoral health and social services systems focused on amelioration of the major causes of ill health, such as poverty and racism.

Although biomedical dominance remains a key driver of the medicalization of oppression, broader systemic forces such as capitalism, globalization, imperialism, neocolonialism and neoliberalism must be integrated into our analysis if we are to continue to change oppressive practices that cause ill health. These broad global forces are central in the resistance to emancipatory ideas about human health. In his discussion of the decline of Canadian left culture, Thom Workman (2009: 16) calls for a renewed left politics that requires "open and reflective discussion, an extensive and exhaustive survey of history, an understanding of the left's past and its unique failures, an analysis of capitalism, an unrelenting commitment to education, a dialogue about the possibilities of change, and the cultivation of strategies covering both the short and the long terms." Workman's call for a healthy left politics reminds us that health must be envisioned, at all levels, to be intimately connected to the social world and to a robust critique of the social origins of ill health.

It is crucial that we reframe health inequities perspectives within the scope of moral responsibility. The central role of addressing public policy-related and ideological origins of ill health must be coupled with a moral compass that directs us to integrate social justice in all aspects of health talk. When families live in chronic poverty, we are morally bound to identify the oppressive public policies that sustain their poverty. For example, in order to move out of poverty, a single mother with one child needs to earn a wage of at least $11 an hour. Most jobs that pay this wage require post-secondary education. According to policy guidelines, single parents on income assistance are not allowed to retain their income assistance benefits while they attend university. A mother attending university cannot pay her tuition and support both herself and her children on a student loan. In the area of Employment Insurance (EI) policy, only 43 percent of unemployed people qualify for EI benefits (NAPO, 2005). Those who do qualify are faced with a two-week un-paid waiting period, which places the poorest and most vulnerable people in real danger. After two weeks an eligible person will receive 55 percent of their earnings averaged over the previous twenty-six weeks.

These numbers mean that a single mother earning minimum wage would have to support herself and her children on a weekly benefit of $167 for fourteen to forty-five weeks, depending upon where she lives. In Halifax, Nova Scotia, this amounts to $2,341 to $7,524. Annually, this amount is $10,028 below Statistics Canada's low income cut-off (LICO) rate for a family of two living in a rural area. Since we know these freely available statistics, are we not morally bound, especially from the relatively privileged positions of policymakers and researchers, to take action and to enhance civil society capacity for action?

It is very discouraging to attend national health conferences, of which I have attended many dozens in Canada, and not hear explicit language of social justice (e.g., oppression, racism, misogyny), or even an occasional nod to the social determinants of health. The lack of this language indicates a relatively superficial treatment of health inequity concerns. Practitioners, researchers and policymakers know that they must add "health inequity" sporadically in their Powerpoint and research funding presentations; however, the presenta-tions themselves, and often the comments and questions from the audience, only occasionally relate to the complex field of critical health studies, where questions about moral responsibility, capitalism and economic globaliza-tion are intimately linked to the health of a nation's citizens. Although the language of the social determinants of health has permeated many provincial and federal health documents, there is scant political commitment to tak-ing aim at the political and economic causes of ill health. This dissonance results in a "having your cake and eating it too" situation for many health and social policymakers and a growing number of health researchers. Inserting the language of inequity (e.g., words such as discrimination, racism, social inequality, social justice) without mirroring the political economy of health inequities (e.g., social murder, taken up in Chapter 2; neoliberalism; neoco-lonialism; imperialism; capitalism; apartheid; systemic oppression) enables policymakers, researchers, educators and research funding bodies to play the SDH game without a consistent commitment to progressive social change.

The environment for critical health studies in Canada is increasingly problematic, particularly in light of recent federal government mandated changes in national research funding policy. The Social Sciences and Humanities Research Council (SSHRC) no longer funds "health" related research, asserting that health should be solely under the purview of the

Canadian Institutes for Health Research (CIHR). This 2009 decision leaves critical health researchers with far less access to research money. Although there has been a dedicated effort on the part of the CIHR to invite social science researchers into their fold, the CIHR's capacity to invite, assess and fund critical health research remains to be demonstrated. Ideas about imperialism, capitalism, social murder and the political economy of health do not easily fit into the rubric of a predominately biomedical funding system. In 2009, the CIHR funded over $425 million in biomedical research, just over $100 million in clinical research, approximately $90 million in population and public health research and just under $50 million in health systems, health services and health policy research (CIHR, 2009). There is thus a significant difference in the funding of biomedical/clinical research and research that is more directly related to SDH concerns ($525 million versus $140 million). Shifting more funding towards the social sciences and the political economy of health inequities will be a considerable fiscal and philosophical challenge.

This edited volume has its genesis in the urgent need to continue to politicize health thinking in Canada and globally. The language of critical analysis is winding its way into mainstream health talk and documentation, but it is often confined to a relatively superficial application of concepts such as equity and diversity. Although there is growing formal acknowledgement of ideas about justice, there is much less admission that justice concepts form a complex field of knowledge in their own right. Rather, it is assumed that policymaking, research, practice and education will somehow honour fairness because commitment to fairness is often considered to be a self-evident truth. This book exemplifies the scope and depth of analysis that must be embraced for progressive social change to truly ameliorate health inequities. We take aim at the causes of the causes of inequities in the social determinants of health in a call for action to put oppression explicitly on the public policy and health and social science research agendas in Canada.

Throughout the book, an anti-oppression framework is used to unravel some of the historical and current pathways that create and sustain health inequities and material and social deprivation. The purpose is to explicitly analyze questions about the structures, processes and systems that have wielded power and to highlight some of the ways that this power must be disrupted. How has it come to be that Aboriginal men have the highest rates of heart disease in Canada? Why do Black women have a much higher rate of death due to cervical cancer compared to White women, despite the fact that Black women have a much lower incidence of that cancer? Why do elder women have the highest rates of depression compared to all other groups? How did it come to be that poverty is the strongest indicator of health status across the lifespan? Why have women's shelters become known as "refugee camps" (Vallee, 2007) for the thousands of women and children who are fleeing from violence in their homes in Canada? We need systemic, critical social scientific answers to these kinds of questions. One of the main contributions of this book is its straightforward commitment to exposing the social, economic and political roots of oppression. The intended audience includes all those who are interested in critical perspectives on health and illness. The chapters provide a core resource for undergraduate and graduate students and educators in a broad range of disciplines and fields, including directly health-related areas (e.g., health and human services, health and human rights, and the political economy of health), as well as sociology and anthropology. This volume is also designed to be relevant for those working "on the ground" with the everyday struggle of health inequities: non-profit agencies such as women's centres and shelters, community health centres and Native friendship centres, shelters for homeless youth and adults, and indeed any practitioners and policymakers who are interested in active solutions to these pressing social problems. Although the book focuses on the Canadian context, it incorporates the global context and, as such, should be of interest to an international audience as well.

Overview of the Book

This book is divided into three sections, and although each chapter has a unique focus, the authors attend to several key linking concepts and issues: systemic power relations and the structural determinants of health, the intersectionality of oppressions with mental and physical health and well-being. Part One, "Politicizing Health," describes how systemic power structures are linked to health. This first chapter provides an overview of the concept of oppression and some of the ways that oppression is related to health across the lifespan. Chapter 2, "People under Threat: Health Outcomes and Oppression," which serves as a linking chapter for the entire book, details the health outcomes of oppression-related stress. Intersectionality is described in terms of its importance for addressing oppression. Although intersectionality theory has been well described elsewhere, I reframe the concept as a synergistic force — one that more aptly describes the dynamic and powerful impacts when the "isms" (e.g., sexism, racism) come together with the SDH and the geographic or spatial contexts of oppression. In Chapter 3, "Critical Perspectives on the Social Determinants of Health," Dennis Raphael draws upon his substantive work in this area to make clear links among the social determinants, health outcomes and the systemic context for the perpetuation of ill health.

Part Two, "How Oppression Operates to Produce Health Inequities," brings the reader into the worlds of those who experience oppression and provides a solid base for understanding the ways that oppression operates in people's everyday lives. In Chapter 4, "Fragmented Performances: Ageism and the Health of Elder Women," Raewyn Bassett discusses oppression as a determinant of women's health from her extensive background in critical sociological perspectives on health. Although critical perspectives on women's health abound, this chapter provides a cohesive portrayal of the specific connections among the oppressions and the health of women. In Chapter 5, "Racism as a Determinant of Health," I join Josephine B. Etowa, an expert in the areas of health inequities and racism and health, to discuss the connections among oppression, racism and the health outcomes of people of colour.

In Chapter 6, "Oppression and the Health of Indigenous Peoples," Marie Battiste and James [Sa'ke'j] Youngblood Henderson draw upon their substantive expertise in the area of Indigenous knowledges and history to present the links among the oppressions of colonialism and neocolonialism and the intergenerational health of Indigenous peoples. In Chapter 7, "Social Exclusion as a Determinant of Health," Grace-Edward Galabuzi integrates his expertise in the area of social exclusion and its powerful impact on everyday life and health. He makes a clear distinction between the use of the terms "social exclusion" and "social inclusion" in order to emphasize the necessary directions for systemic change. Chapter 8, "Oppression and Im/migrant Health," discusses the area of immigrant and migrant health. Denise Spitzer draws upon her expertise in the area of gender, migration and health to explore the historical and current systemic context of the health of immigrants. In Chapter 9, "Oppression and Mental Health: Pathologizing Injustice," I draw upon mental health and community clinical practice and academic work to detail the power of oppression to shape mental health. The chapter particularly underscores the need for social change to interrogate the relationship between psychiatrization and oppression.

Part Three, "Toward Structural Change," builds on the social change focus of the previous sections. In Chapter 10, Oppression, Health and Public Policy in Canada, Toba Bryant builds on her expertise in the area of public policy and health to discuss some of the systemic foundations of oppression. In Chapter 11, "Tackling Oppression with a Human Rights-Based Approach to Primary Health Care Renewal," Charmaine McPherson draws on her expertise in the area of primary health care renewal and reform in a call for a human rights-based approach to re-shaping primary health care from a global perspective. . In Chapter 12, "The Political Economy of Health Inequities," I join Lars K. Hallstrom in a discussion of the importance of understanding the political economy of health if we are to achieve equity in health outcomes. Chapter 13, "Health as a Human Right: Challenges and Practical Applications," concludes the book with an emphasis on the morally indefensible actions and inactions that create and sustain health inequities. I join Maureen Shebib, a lawyer who has worked extensively in the area of human rights, equity and discrimination, to discuss the connections between health and human rights.

Defining Oppression

The concept of oppression has long been an important consideration for social scientists and others interested in the amelioration of social injustice. The interconnected mechanisms of oppression bear many temporal and spatial similarities. They include genocide, cultural genocide, policy-created poverty, dangerous work environments, and numerous actions and inactions that create and maintain systems of dominance. At the heart of oppression is structural power. While individuals can exert social and cultural power over other individuals, it is structural power in national and global systems, such as education, governance, law and health, that cements and sustains oppression across time and across earth's geographies. The cycle of oppression, described in more detail below, shows how individual acts of stereotyping and discrimination are integral in creating and sustaining systemic oppression. As Iris Marion Young (1990: 41) tells us, oppression refers to "the vast and deep injustices some groups suffer as a consequence of often unconscious assumptions and reactions of well-meaning people in ordinary interactions, media and cultural stereotypes, and structural features of bureaucratic hierarchies and market mechanisms — in short, the normal processes of everyday life."

Young's description reminds us of the embedded nature of oppression and the central importance of unpacking the ways that oppression is linked to power relations. Power, in this sense, is not a static entity or a thing, but rather it is best understood as relational. While the exercise of power may depend on certain material resources, such as money, military equipment, and so on, these resources should not be confused with power itself (Young, 1990). For example, in health care systems, governing structures wield considerable power over the implementation of policies for the allocation of material and human resources, such as money, health clinics and health care workers. Manipulation of these resources is possible through various kinds of power, including political and economic power.

In Canada the deterioration of the principles of the *Canada Health Act, 1984*, is a living example of the ways that different kinds of power may be used to sustain oppression. Although the Act is ostensibly enshrined in, or protected by, our legal system, power relations are involved in at least two key oppressive practices: 1) active maintenance, through consistent action and inaction, of a system of barriers that create limited health care access for many Canadians, including Indigenous people, persons with disabilities and families who live in poverty; and 2) the deterioration of publicly funded health care through consistent promotion of a privately funded, market-driven system. Power relations involved in the maintenance of limited health care access include institutional (e.g., government, health system) practices of assuming that families have the means to obtain transportation and child care to attend health care appointments and the money to buy a vast range of supplementary treatments, such as over-the-counter antibiotic creams, orthotic shoe inserts, special bandages for home care after surgery, sunscreen, vitamins and supplements, hot and cold packs for treatment of chronic pain — the list is potentially endless. Barriers in access also originate in insufficient action in the education and health care systems regarding the integration of principles of cultural safety in policy and practice. Power relations involved in the movement to privatize health care include an array of market-driven interests that seek to create a for-profit health care system — an approach that has been shown to undermine the effectiveness and inherent justice of universal, accessible, publicly funded health care. These two examples illustrate that oppressive power relations often operate through inaction. Few provincial governments in Canada, and certainly not the federal government, would agree that they are actively promoting privatization. However, government and legal system inaction, and in some cases active support of privatization, in the face of growing corporate domination of health care in Canada, constitutes active participation in these oppressive practices.

Since such power relations exercise dominance in shifting health care in a particular direction, they are also referred to as ruling relations (McGibbon, 2004). Dorothy Smith describes ruling relations as "a complex of organized practices, including government, law, business and financial management, professional organizations, and educational institutions as well as the discourses and texts that interpenetrate the multiple sites of power" (1987: 3). These relations of ruling organize and regulate our lives in contemporary society (Smith, 2005). One of the reasons that oppression is difficult to grasp is that it happens in a fluid and dynamic way, and its mechanisms of action and inaction are not clearly visible. Oppression becomes most visible when resistance movements expose the harsh everyday realities of structural power and actively fight for the rights of oppressed peoples and groups.

An Example: The Oppression of Women

The struggles for women's enfranchisement provide a concrete example of how oppression and resistance to oppression may come about. In keeping with the structural and policy-based mechanisms of oppression, denying suffrage to Canadian women was enshrined in the Constitution of Canada. White women won the right to vote in elections in 1918, but they were not recognized as persons until 1929. Canadian women of Asian and Indo-Canadian heritage were not enfranchised until 1947. Indigenous women could not vote until 1960. These facts illustrate one of the key features of oppression, namely that it does not operate in isolation. As the disenfranchisement of Indigenous, Asian, and Indo-Canadian women demonstrates, the oppressions of sexism and racism form a powerful synergy in disadvantaging women of colour in Canada.

A related key aspect of oppression is that ruling relations and those who support them will not easily give up power. Each of these waves of enfranchisement for women was won through well organized political lobbying, public demonstrations and a host of other consciousness-raising actions directed at achieving justice in the face of oppression. The legal and government system did not "give" the vote to White women, or subsequently to Asian, Indo-Canadian and Indigenous women. Enfranchisement was the result of relentless action on the part of women and their allies and was consistently dovetailed with state-based physical and verbal violence against women, as evidenced by the beating and incarceration of many women during the suffragist movement in England in the 1800s.

There are many other examples of the positive results of active resistance to the oppression of women in Canada. In 1969 the dissemination of birth control information was decriminalized; in 1974 the remaining overt discrimination against female immigrants was removed from the *Citizenship Act*; in 1978 the Canadian Labour Code was amended to prohibit dismissal or layoff because of pregnancy; in 1981 women's rights were included in the Canadian Constitution; in 1985 the *Indian Act* was amended to restore status to First Nations women who were married to non-status men; and in 1993 refugee guidelines were amended to include women facing gender-based persecution. Each of these accomplishments was won through decades of arduous pressure against dominant power structures, such as the Canadian government and the legal system in local, provincial and national arenas. These examples provide everyday meaning about how oppression unfolds and point to the all-encompassing impact of oppression on people's lives and health. The oppression of women meant that they could not own property; they could not obtain birth control information without threat of fines or imprisonment as recently as 1969; they did not have the legal rights of citizens, including protection under the law; and they could not formally participate in state governing of any kind.

These profound barriers to participation and protection exemplify how oppression might have lasting and intergenerational impacts on everyday life and health. Although there is increasing attention to the health impacts of social inequities, the movement to link social, political and economic circumstance to the health of citizens is relatively recent. Authors such as Marmot and Wilkinson (1999) and Raphael (2006, 2009a) have developed the now well-recognized framework of the social determinants of health to stress the social, political and economic antecedents of poor health outcomes. The gaze is now shifting from individual biologic and genetic endowment and "lifestyle" to oppressive, policy-entrenched inequities that create and sustain poor health outcomes in communities and across generations. The importance of biology and genetics notwithstanding, the problem has been, and continues to be, that an individualistic focus dominates public-policy creation and implementation at the expense of the health of citizens.

The Cycle of Oppression

The following section describes the cycle of oppression. I discuss the links between everyday bias and stereotyping, and oppression. Although systemic oppression is the focus of each of the chapters in this volume, it is crucial to ground oppression in the day-to-day and relentless bias and stereotyping that forms its substrate. This approach also reminds us that oppression, while a systemic force, is activated and perpetuated through human relationships — the collective ways that we treat each other as individuals, communities, and nations.

It is very difficult to explore oppression because it is a complex process, rather than a discrete event. Ideas about domination, power and discrimination are interconnected, and there are many different and synergistic kinds of oppressions. These include sexism, racism, heterosexism, ableism, ageism and classism, to name a few. The "isms" refer to the use of systemic power to deny people access to resources, rights, respect and representation on the basis of age, culture, ethnicity, gender, income, nationality, race, religion, sexuality, social class, spirituality or membership in any other group (McGibbon & Etowa, 2009). Oppression embeds itself in everyday life through a cyclic process involving biased information and stereotyping, prejudice, discrimination and oppression. Although the representation of the cycle of oppression presented in Figure 1.1 may somewhat simplify this complex process, it nonetheless provides a concrete way to bring theoretical ideas into

Figure 1.1 Ruling Power Relations and the Cycle of Oppression

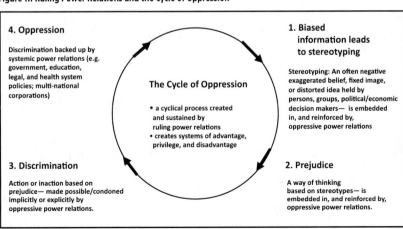

Source: *Adapted from McGibbon, Etowa & McPherson, 2008a.*

the world of everyday lived experience — a process that is urgently needed if we are to confront oppressive practices that cause ill health. We must find a way to bring the language of critical social science to the kitchen tables, staff room tables, boardroom tables and research conference tables across Canada and globally.

As Toba Bryant describes in Chapter 10, oppression is both a state and a process (Prilletensky & Gonick, 1996). Oppression as a state or outcome happens through the consistent denial of access to resources, resulting in deprivation, exclusion, discrimination and exploitation (Prilletensky & Gonick 1996; Sidanius, 1993). Oppression as a process involves institutionalized procedures and practices of domination and control. The oppression of Indigenous peoples around the globe serves as an urgently important example of how this process operates over time.

Biased Information and Stereotyping

Biased information about Indigenous peoples has a strong historical foundation that remains difficult to disrupt. Colonization implants a way of thinking about people and relationships among people that sets up hierarchal dualisms and oppressive values, beliefs and assumptions based on identities such as race, gender, religion and ethnicity. Over time, these values and beliefs are assumed to be correct and are passed on through institutional practices from childrearing to schooling, to professional socialization and ultimately to national policy (McGibbon, Didham, Smith, Malaudzi, & Barton, 2009). Although there are many innovative education programs that teach about Indigenous history and lifeways, very little factual information is mandated for explicit curriculum inclusion in Canadian schools, in post-secondary education and in education of the public in general.

Although there is ample evidence of the centuries-long brutal treatment and genocide of Indigenous peoples at the hands of European colonizers, these details remain largely unknown to most Canadians. We have barely begun to engage in the truth and reconciliation process that is surely a moral imperative for Canada. In the absence of access to documented historical evidence and first-voice accounts of the impact of imperialism, colonization and re-colonization, Canadians are immersed in biased information that leads to stereotyping about Indigenous peoples. Stereotypes are maintained over time by policies and lack of policies, as is the case in the Canadian government's lack of action regarding establishing a truth and reconciliation process.

> The destruction of every civilization that thrived in the Americas, and the annihilation of 70–100 million Indigenous souls during the European invasion speaks for itself. These assaults, committed against innocent people in the name of greed, mean that each modern nation in the Americas was founded with the spilling of

much Native American blood. Consequently, there can be no real peace in the Americas until each European-founded nation assumes responsibility for past crimes against humanity and makes atonement to Native Americans for the indescribable horrors to which they subjected them. (Paul, 2006, p. 1)

Dr. Daniel Paul's words remind us of the urgent need to educate Canadians about Indigenous genocide in order to disrupt the persistent flow of biased information and hence stereotyping of Indigenous peoples. One way to think about a stereotype is that it is like a fixed image. It is an exaggerated belief, image or distorted idea held by persons, groups and political and economic decision-makers, to name a few. It is a generalization that allows for little or no individual difference or social variation (McGibbon & Etowa, 2009). Chapter 5 describes some of the common cultural stereotypes of Aboriginal, Black and Asian Canadians. A particularly persistent and odious stereotype that many White people continue to have about Indigenous people is that they are lazy and do not want to work. This stereotype has its roots in European colonization, where these kinds of beliefs were promoted by power relations in government and education through mechanisms such as the media of the day (e.g., posters, pamphlets) and to Indigenous peoples themselves through many other processes, such as the Indian residential school system. The continued perpetuation of stereotypes of Indigenous peoples, along with myriad other processes, creates an intricate system of modern-day re-colonization.

Prejudice
Stereotypes lead to a particular way of thinking and attitudes that are prejudiced. Prejudice literally means to "pre-judge." A common and persistent prejudice that White people hold about Indigenous people in Canada is that they "have had everything given to them and still can't live well, or work and be healthy — free houses, free tuition, extra tax breaks, etc." Here we see the direct links among biased information, stereotyping and prejudice. Without knowledge, or even acknowledgement, of the brutal mechanisms of colonization and re-colonization, how can Canadians understand the powerful impact of colonialism's intergenerational traumatization and the folly of thinking that occasional housing subsidies and augmented university tuition for some Indigenous people will undo history? The very persistence of these distorted ideas is evidence of successful systemic reinforcement of prejudicial thinking over time. These concerns are further taken up by Marie Battiste and James [Sa'ke'j] Youngblood Henderson in Chapter 7.

Discrimination

Discrimination is action or inaction based on prejudice. Although individuals can discriminate, these individual social relations are organized and coordinated by a set of ruling relations beyond individual acts of discrimination. These extra-local power relations create the foundation upon which discrimination can flourish. It is important to note that these external controls are not always visible within the local experience (McGibbon, 2004). For example, studies show that health care professionals consistently discriminate against Indigenous and Black people and their families (McGibbon & Etowa, 2009). The clinicians who are perpetrating this discrimination are not likely to identify their individual lack of action as discriminatory, nor are they likely to identify that they are practising within a system of ruling relations that condones their individual discrimination. Discrimination is created, re-created and reinforced by power relations. The health care, education and legal systems continue to be instrumental in this process.

The Canadian Criminal Justice Association (CCJA, 2000) has documented numerous examples: compared to Caucasian Canadians, Aboriginal people who are accused of a crime are more likely to be denied bail and more likely to be charged with multiple offences, often for crimes against the system; more time is spent in pre-trial detention by Aboriginal people; Aboriginal people are more likely not to have legal representation at court proceedings; Aboriginal clients, especially in Northern communities where the court party flies in on the day of the hearing, spend less time with their lawyers; Aboriginal offenders are more than twice as likely to be incarcerated; and in all institutions, Aboriginal Elders, who are also spiritual leaders, are not given the same status as prison priests and chaplains (CCJA). These acts of discrimination against Aboriginal people are made possible through the support of systemic power.

Oppression

Oppression is discrimination backed up by systemic or structural power, sometimes referred to as institutionalized power, including government, education, legal and health system policies and practices. Following from the previous examples, the perpetuation of stereotypes about Indigenous peoples is made possible, as Smith (1987) notes, through a complex of organized practices, including health care systems that condone discrimination, professional associations that fail to hold clinicians accountable for their well-documented discriminatory practices and professional education institutions that consistently fail to prepare clinicians with adequate knowledge of the critical social science of health inequities. Oppressive practices in government and law are articulated to these health system practices to produce a well-organized system of oppression that becomes inscribed on the bodies and spirits of Indigenous peoples.

The cycle of oppression thus underscores the chain of causation in oppressive practices that leads us squarely to focus on the systemic causes of ill health — the causes of the causes. Since oppression, by definition, is deeply embedded in systemic ruling relations, the results of oppression are persistent and toxic for the mental, physical and spiritual health of oppressed people. Health outcomes of oppressed people are alarmingly worse when compared to Canadian averages (see Chapter 2 for numerous examples). The cycle of oppression illustrates that oppression feeds on itself to produce increasing social and material deprivation and hardship and, ultimately, increasingly worse health outcomes. Systemic oppression reinforces existing biases and stereotypes while creating new variations that result in a compounding of oppressions.

Tackling the social determinants of health is an increasingly important social imperative in Canada and globally. There has been a gradual evolution from viewing the SDH as somewhat self evident (of course lack of education will result in lower incomes) to viewing inequities in the SDH as direct consequences of systemic inequities. Individuals, families and communities are under increasing threat of poor health, and in particular the threat of policies that increase the social and material deprivation that characterizes poverty. This latter way of thinking about the SDH also carries a moral imperative for social change. It is no longer sufficient for researchers, policymakers and practitioners to philosophically support the idea of systemic change while confining their actions to the realm of the status quo.

2

People under Threat

Health Outcomes and Oppression

Elizabeth A. McGibbon

When one individual inflicts bodily injury upon another such that death results, we call the deed manslaughter; when the assailant knew in advance that the injury would be fatal, we call this deed murder. But when society places hundreds of proletarians in such a position that they inevitably meet a too early and an unnatural death, one which is quite as much a death by violence as a sword or a bullet; when it deprives thousands of the necessities of life, places them under conditions in which they cannot live — forces them, through the strong arm of the law, to remain in such conditions until that death ensues, which is the inevitable consequence — knows that these thousands of victims must perish, yet permits these conditions to remain, its deed is murder just as surely as the deed of the single individual; disguised malicious murder, murder against which none can defend himself, which does not seem what it is, because no man sees the murderer, because the death of the victim seems a natural one, since the offence is more one of omission than commission. But murder it remains. (Engels, 2009 [1845]: 152)

This chapter discusses some of the ways that oppression is inscribed on body and mind. I reframe the concept of "vulnerable people" and "people at risk" to "people under threat" as a way to focus attention on the causes of the causes of social and material deprivation and ill health. Health outcomes of oppression-related stress are detailed in terms of mental (psychological and spiritual) and physical (physical and physiological) processes. The synergies of oppression-related stress are described, including the ways that mental stress interacts with physical and physiological stress. Building on previous work (McGibbon, 2009), I describe intersections of social determinants of health (SDH) related oppression. Intersectionality theory is extended to incorporate intersections of the SDH, the isms as SDH (racism, sexism, classism, etc) and geography as an SDH. The chronic health conditions of asthma and juvenile rheumatoid arthritis are highlighted within the frame of intersectionality.

Reframing "Vulnerable People" as "People under Threat"

The discourse of health inequalities and inequities commonly refers to "vulnerable people" in an attempt to identify those who are particularly "at risk." However, if we are committed to tackling oppression-related health outcomes, it is incumbent upon us to reframe the concept of vulnerable people to "people under threat." The vulnerability discourse implies that an individual or community is somehow more prone to experiencing health inequities, in much the same way as one might be prone to catching a cold. The concept of vulnerability worked well when it first came into common usage because it allowed us to name the people who are most oppressed and thereby attempt to influence public policy in the direction of justice. However, the term is not ultimately effective in ameliorating the physical, spiritual and psychological suffering caused by injustice because it reinforces the idea of a nebulous force that is somehow causing ill health. Rather, it is time to reframe our thinking to explicitly identify the threats that are causing ill health: colonization, re-colonization, post-colonialism, neoliberal economic policy and corporatization of health care delivery, to name a few.

Yes, people are certainly vulnerable; however, our task is to identify the social pathogens that threaten health. We must answer the question: What and who are creating these risks for "at risk" people? This chapter emphasizes these systemic risks and their impact on body, mind and community — the modern-day social murder that causes certain groups to persistently suffer more and to die earlier. Engels' words of 1844 were eerily prophetic for Canadians today who are passionate about moving the anti-oppression project forward: citizens meeting too early and unnatural deaths, health and public-policy systems depriving thousands of the necessities of life, and knowing that thousands must perish, yet permitting such conditions to remain. The measure of a society is its willingness to provide for the collective well-being of all citizens, especially those who are most under threat of social and material deprivation. Countries such as Sweden have demonstrated to the world that social democratic public policy supports health for all, along with a strong, fiscally responsible economy. These facts demonstrate that ill health is tied to a nation's political will to make (or not to make) socially just policy decisions over time.

How Oppression Is Inscribed on Body and Mind

"We take it as a basic fact that we all live and act in bodies that literally embody — biologically, across the lifecourse — our societal and ecological context" (Krieger, 2005, p. 8). The social consequences of oppression have been brought forward by numerous social activists and scholars, including Patricia Hill Collins (1990), Franz Fanon (1963) and Edward Said (1979).

Chapter 1 describes how oppression causes social disruption, intergenerational traumatization and profound psychological, spiritual and mental suffering. For example, oppression through displacement or translocation creates loss of family land, homes and communal property and ultimately results in a deep disruption of culture, spirituality and language. Oppression of workers, through practices such as maintaining unsafe working conditions and unfair remuneration, also happens around the globe. Ultimately, these oppressions create threats of intergenerational poverty that remain exceedingly difficult to disrupt.

Although the social consequences of oppression have been theorized for decades, drawing explicit links between oppressive social circumstances and longitudinal evidence about the health outcomes of oppressed peoples has barely begun. Still today, when we as a society ask ourselves questions such as why certain groups (e.g., women, persons with a disability, Indigenous people, African Canadians) earn less money than the average Canadian, we turn to their lack of education as a reason. True, lack of education is a strong predictor of lack of employment success. But why do these groups persistently have less education? Because their families could not afford to send them to school. But why is it that their families could not afford to send them to school? Because their parents didn't have adequate employment. But why didn't they have adequate employment? Because they could not go to school. These questions illustrate the circular reasoning that results when we confine our attention to an individualistic focus. In this micro realm, we cannot come to grips with the systemic causes of poverty and hence the systemic causes of ill health. These systemic causes are also known as the structural determinants of health. As described in Chapter 12, they are called structural because "they are part of the political, economic, and social structure of society and of the culture that informs them" (Navarro, 2007a. p. 2). Emphasis is directed to the role of the economic organization of society in the production and distribution of disease and burden of illness and to the ways that disease and illness are framed and treated (McGibbon, 2009).

Oppression encompasses these structural determinants of health, and it creates and sustains the chronic physical and psychological stress that ultimately leads to persistent physical and mental health problems. Although this phenomenon may seem self-evident, the mechanisms that are operating are not often scrutinized and are scarcely integrated into health and human service assessment and intervention or health and social policy. Numerous studies have shown that certain groups of people experience consistent discrimination based on their gender, social class, race, ethnicity, age and sexual orientation and so on (Duncan & Lorreto, 2004; Fish, 2007; Karlsen & Nazroo, 2002), and evidence demonstrates that people living in poverty, women, elders, people of colour and lesbian, gay and bisexual people have

Figure 2.1 People under Threat: Health Outcomes and Oppression

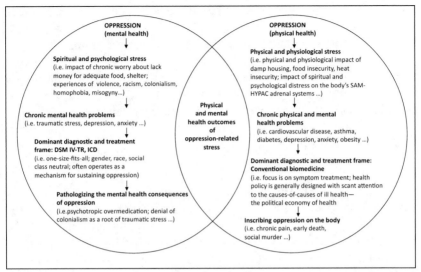

poorer health outcomes (McGibbon, 2009). The threat of oppression, and oppression itself, has a persistent impact on mental and physical health, and these two aspects of stress do not happen in isolation. Rather, they happen together to produce a powerful synergy that is ultimately inscribed on the bodies and minds of oppressed peoples.

Figure 2.1 illustrates this synergy. Spiritual and psychological stress often leads to chronic mental health problems. In Western countries, these struggles are most often categorized under the psychiatric rubric of the *Diagnostic and Statistical Manual of Mental Disorders* (American Psychiatric Association, 2004) or the International Classification of Diseases ([ICD-10] WHO, 2007d). Chapter 9 of this volume describes how this process leads to pathologizing the mental health consequences of oppression. Individual psychiatric diagnoses and individual-based treatment, often with psychotropic medications, does little to address the persistent structural causes of depression, post-traumatic stress and anxiety.

Along with psychological and spiritual stress, oppressed people experience physical and physiological stress. The dominant treatment frame in Western countries is conventional biomedicine, where treatment remains focused on the individual and on individual body systems and parts. This individual-based focus perpetuates the inscription of oppression on body and mind. Figure 2.1 describes these processes. Note that mental health is an integral aspect of both sides of the diagram.

The Spiritual and Psychological Stress of Oppression

Spiritual and psychological stresses are core aspects of oppression. Key features of these stresses are briefly described here to underscore their synergistic relationship with the physical and physiological stresses of oppression. As Figure 2.1 illustrates, mental health consequences of oppression have two pathways. The more recognized pathway involves chronic mental health problems resulting from persistent spiritual and psychological distress. The less acknowledged pathway involves chronic mental health problems resulting from persistent distress on the body's adrenal system — the stress-handling system. Chapter 9 provides a detailed description of the spiritual and psychological stress of oppression.

The Physical and Physiological Stress of Oppression

Physical and physiological outcomes of oppression continue to be consistently borne out in the health outcomes of citizens. The psychological and spiritual stress of chronic worrying about basic necessities such as food and shelter happen concurrently with all the associated bodily stresses. These stresses are the embodiment of poverty across the lifespan. The physical impacts of damp housing and heat and food insecurity are well documented. The asthma epidemic in North America and the United Kingdom, among other areas, has been clearly linked to substandard housing and proximity to crowded urban centres. Children living in damp and mouldy dwellings have a greater prevalence of respiratory symptoms, including wheezing, sore throats and runny noses, as well as headaches and fever, compared to children in dry houses (Beasley, Masoli, Fabian, and Holt, 2004; Shelter Cymru, 2004).

People with asthma are more than twice as likely to live in damp houses. Low housing temperatures have been shown to lower resistance to respiratory infections, damp housing leads to mould growth and fungi, which can cause allergies and respiratory infections, and cold impairs lung function and can trigger broncho-constriction and asthma (Beasley, Masoli, Fabian, and Holt, 2004; Shelter Cymru, 2004). In a European study of 6,683 urban children, childhood asthma and allergic rhinitis were positively correlated with exposure to major urban air pollutants (Penard-Morand, Raherison, Charpin, et al., 2010). In North America, studies have shown that individuals with asthma living in areas with high ozone and particulate pollution levels are more likely to have frequent asthma symptoms and asthma-related emergency department visits and hospitalizations (Meng, Rull, Wilhelm, et al., 2010).

Heat insecurity has an impact on a growing number of households because poverty has placed these families in a "heat or eat" crisis. In the United States, the National Energy Assistance Directors' Association (NEADA, 2008) completed its first national survey of utility averages and utility shut-offs in 2008. Based on a sample of eleven states representing 25 percent of all households, an estimated 1.2 million households were disconnected from electric and natural gas service from March through May, following the expiration of state shut-off moratoria. On average, these families owed about $850 in past-due utility bills, with the total amount exceeding $1 billion. The number of families who endure shut-offs is likely to rise as utilities continue credit and collection procedures related to the end-of-winter shut-off moratoria (NEADA, 2008; Presser, 2008).

Food insecurity is a growing social concern in Canada (Tarusuk, 2005). Families and individuals who lack food security experience uncertainty that they will be able to acquire and consume adequate quality and quantity of food in mainstream ways; consume nutritionally inadequate food; consume reduced quantity and quality of food; and acquire and consume food in non-mainstream (socially unacceptable) ways or by incurring further disadvantage (depleting assets, not spending on necessary medications, etc.) (Rainville & Brink, 2001). According to Tarusuk (2005), food insecurity was recognized as a problem in Canada in the early 1980s, when community groups began to establish charitable food assistance programs in response to concerns that people in their midst were going hungry. Since then, the number of Canadians affected by food insecurity has steadily grown.

In 1998, approximately 3 million respondents, approximately 10.2 percent of the population in Canada, lived in a household that experienced an episode of food insecurity in the past year. The proportion of respondents who were children was higher (13.4 percent) than respondents who were adults (9.3 percent). Most of these food insecure households were food anxious (e.g., worried about how they will acquire their next meal) (8 percent) or compromised their diet (7.8 percent). About 4 percent of Canadians, or 1.2 million, experienced an episode in the last year when they or someone in their household did not have enough food to eat because of a lack of money (Rainville & Brink, 2001). In a study of food insecurity and hunger among 141 low-income lone mothers with children in Atlantic Canada, 96.5 percent experienced food insecurity over the previous year (McIntyre, Glanville, Officer, et al., 2002).

> But food charity remains the primary response. Children's feeding programs, prenatal nutrition programs, and a number of smaller scale, community development programs have also been instituted. However, growing recognition of the limitations of these efforts to address food problems rooted in chronically inadequate household incomes has led to a renewed emphasis on advocacy for social policy reforms. (Tarusuk, 2005, p. 299)

These physical stresses, of course, happen in tandem with the spiritual and psychological stresses of chronic worry about food, shelter and heating the family home in the cold Canadian winter. These worries, along with the stresses of everyday racism, sexism, homophobia and the impacts of colonialism have a profound impact on the body's stress managing systems — the sympathetic adrenal medulla (SAM) and the hypothalamus-pituitary-adrenal cortex (HYPAC), both located near the brain. The SAM-HYPAC system is structured to deal with everyday stresses in addition to more acute stresses. The system regulates our bodies through short-term stressful times and helps us maintain overall wellness. The problem arises when long-term, chronic stresses, such as those described above, eventually overtax the SAM-HYPAC system. The adrenal system becomes overwhelmed and is unable to maintain physiological balance. The result is adrenal fatigue. Chronic adrenal fatigue causes depression, obesity, hypertension, diabetes, cancer, ulcers, chronic stomach problems, allergies and eczema, autoimmune diseases, headaches, kidney and liver disease, and overall reduced immunity (Varcarolis, 2008). These physical and mental health outcomes of adrenal fatigue are embodied in oppressed peoples. They combine with social and material deprivation and discrimination to create consistently unjust health outcomes and an everyday kind of physical and spiritual suffering that has gone unacknowledged for far too long.

The health care system is ill-equipped to engage in the anti-oppressive practice necessary to honour the impact of chronic stress on the minds and bodies of oppressed individuals and families. While deprivations such as food insecurity cause low-income families to eat foods that increase obesity and heart disease, chronic oppression-related stress in the body's adrenal system also contributes heavily to these compromised health outcomes. This is why new terms such as "obesogenic" environments, a renewed focus on "lifestyle choices" and millions of research dollars being poured into linking obesity with individual shortcomings, such as lack of exercise, are an affront to those who experience systemic forms of oppression. The lifestyle rhetoric thus frames the outcomes of oppression as a personal "choice." While exercise and diet are certainly important, a focus on these factors reinforces an ultimately fruitless individualistic approach to health problems that have their origins in the causes of the causes of ill health. Popular culture and at times governments themselves sustain threatening stereotypes about oppressed peoples, such as homeless youth ("they are on the street because they don't like the rules at home," despite robust evidence linking policy-created poverty with family hardship) and social assistance recipients ("they are all lazy welfare bums," despite the fact that most social assistance recipients in Canada are lone mothers). The following paragraphs detail some of these oppression-related health outcomes.

First Nations peoples living on reserves have reported rates of heart diseases four times higher than the overall Canadian rate (HSF, 2009) and First

Nations women and men have life expectancies 5.3 and 7.4 years shorter, respectively, than Canadians as a whole (Health Canada, 2003). Chronic and infectious disease rates are higher in Indigenous (First Nations, Inuit and Métis) peoples on and off reserve than in non-Indigenous Canadians: arthritis and rheumatism (26 percent for Indigenous peoples, 16 percent for non-Indigenous); high blood pressure (15 percent versus 13 percent); and tuberculosis rate per 100,000/year (21 percent versus 1.3 percent) (CIHI, 2004). Ethnic minority women are diagnosed with more advanced breast cancer and experience greater morbidity and mortality (Kimlin, Padilla, & Tejero, 2004).

First Nations adults in Canada have a 20.8 percent higher rate of cancer than the general Canadian population (Assembly of First Nations, 2007). African American men have a much higher risk of prostate cancer, a higher-grade disease at diagnosis and a higher mortality and morbidity rate than Caucasian men (Maliski, Connor, Fink, et al., 2006). In a study by Quan, Fong, De Coster, et al. (2006), members of visible minorities were found to be less likely to be admitted to hospital or tested for a prostate-specific antigen as a screen for prostate cancer, administered a mammogram (breast cancer screening) or given a pap test (cervical cancer screening). African-Americans were more likely than Whites to report that they felt discriminated against in their ability to obtain care or treatment for their pain because of race or ethnicity (Whites 9 percent, African-Americans 15 percent, Hispanics 13 percent). This difference became far larger, however, when the focus was on males with low income (family incomes less than $25,000). In this subgroup, African-Americans were almost three times as likely as Whites to feel they have been discriminated against in their efforts to obtain treatment for pain (27 percent versus 10 percent) (Nguyenlo, Ugarte, Fuller, et al., 2005).

The dominant diagnostic and treatment frame for mental and physical health struggles in the West is conventional biomedicine. Efforts to engage in a more "holistic" approach notwithstanding, the focus is still predominately on symptom management. Although some practitioners, especially those working in non-profit agencies and community development-based health centres, work within a social scientific model of care, the vast majority of health interventions in Canada remain rooted in the biomedical approach of physical and mental symptom assessment and "evidence-based" intervention. In Canada, a resurgence of interest in the renewal of primary health care holds great promise for shifting the focus of health care towards the principles in the Declaration of the Alma Ata (WHO, 1978). The Alma Ata affirmed that health care should be rooted in universal, community-based, preventive and curative services with substantial community involvement and inclusion of nurses and health extension officers who would be educated to work in community health centres. Chapter 11 further explores the Alma Ata in the context of primary health care.

Oppressive practices, including the stereotyping, prejudice and discrimination that underpin systemic oppression, combine to create a vast array of deep and persistent health problems. As the above evidence shows, the complexity of how these oppressions operate is further reinforced by their intersectionality. It is not possible to comprehend oppressions related to disability, poverty and racism without locating sexism as a contributing oppression, thus underscoring that oppressions operate as a complex system.

Synergies of Oppression:
A Framework for Tackling SDH Inequities

The concept of oppression does not lend itself to practical application, which is one reason why it has taken so long to make explicit linkages between the processes of oppression and their impact on health. This section makes some of these linkages and paths to social action more clear through the use of an intersectionality lens for tackling SDH health inequities. Intersectionality theory details the interaction of the impacts of various forms of oppression related to the "isms" and the links among the oppressions and systemic power (Calliste & Dei, 2000; Collins, 1990; Anderson & Collins, 2007). These forms of discrimination, and hence oppression, in society do not operate independently of each other. Rather, they interact in a complex manner that intensifies oppression. Descriptors of oppression such as intersecting and interlocking bring the discussion beyond additive models, which fail to stress the centrality of power and privilege (Collins, 1990). An intersectionality framework has been used to describe the interwoven influences of identities such as gender, sexual orientation, race, ethnicity, disability and age on experiences of injustice (James, 1996; Calliste & Dei, 2000). Feminist intersectionality frameworks emphasize "an understanding of the many circumstances that combine with discriminatory social practices to produce and sustain inequity and exclusion. Intersectional feminist frameworks look at how systems of discrimination such as colonialism and globalization can impact the combination of a person's social or economic status, race, class, gender, and sexuality" (CRIAW, 2006, p. 7).

Intersectionality is beginning to be explicitly incorporated into discussions about the social determinants of health and women's health research (McGibbon & Etowa, 2007, 2009; Hankivsky & Christoffersen, 2008; Hankivsky & Cormier, 2010; Hankivsky, Cormier, & de Merich, 2009), and primary health care renewal (McPherson & McGibbon, 2010b). Figure 2.2 builds on earlier work (McGibbon, 2007, 2009) in an effort to design a practical model that allows for multiple intersections, including, but not limited to, the "isms." Although the concept of intersectionality is key in understanding the health impacts of oppression, it falls somewhat short when one considers how the isms, the SDH and geography all combine in a deadly synergy for oppressed peoples. These three areas must be woven together to enrich an understanding of paths for policy and civil society action to reduce health inequities: (1) identity and the "isms" (e.g., racism, sexism, classism) as SDH, (2) the SDH as laid out in the Toronto Charter (Raphael, 2009a), as revised by Mikkonen and Raphael (2010) and (3) geography as an SDH.

Already there has been a merging of the first two areas (the isms and the SDH) because some of the "isms" are sometimes referred to as SDH (e.g., race/racism and gender/sexism). However, all of the isms, as the evidence in this chapter shows, are also determinants of health. The geographic or spatial contexts of oppression introduce another layer of complexity, including rural and remote lack of access to services, and the persistent location of toxic waste sites close to communities of colour (McGibbon & Etowa, 2007). Chapter 5 provides more details about environmental racism and its structural, policy-based supports.

When we consider the spatial contexts of oppression along with the

Figure 2.2 Synergies of Oppression: An Intersectionality Framework for Tackling SDH Inequities

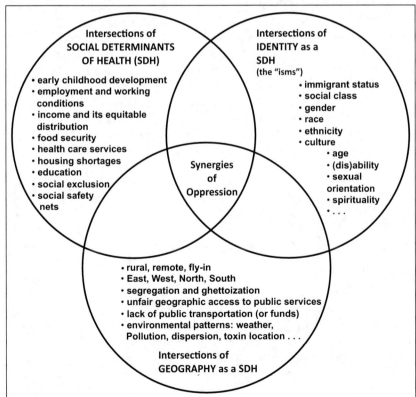

Box 2.1 Intersectionality and Chronic Illness in Canada

Marya is seven years old. She has recently been diagnosed with juvenile rheumatoid arthritis (JRA), an autoimmune condition which causes, among other problems, painful and possibly deforming swelling in her joints, particularly her ankles, wrists and knees. Her family lives in a rural area where there are no clinicians with expertise in rheumatology, or its sub-specialty, JRA. The nearest pediatric rheumatologist is a two and a half hour drive away. Appointments are routinely booked without consultation regarding family availability, and cancelling an appointment results in delays of up to six months for another appointment, even if Marya's condition worsens. Mom works as a cashier at a large supermarket ($9/hr), and dad works as a carpenter ($23/hr). His work is seasonal. Since the family must travel to the city for an appointment, one of the parents must negotiate a full day off work, thus losing a day's pay (average $120 lost wages). Marya also has other autoimmune conditions, and her long-term prognosis remains precarious and thus very worrisome for her parents. The family has a car, but it is only used for local travel dues to its condition. They borrow a neighbour's car (gas and mileage = $210 return). Even though the neighbours will not charge mileage, the material cost is still incurred.

The appointment with the rheumatologist happens in tandem with other specialist appointments with an occupational therapist and a physiotherapist. At the occupational therapy appointment, the therapist fits Marya with special support braces for her wrists. *After* the fitting and moulding of the braces is complete, the parents are told that they must pay for the braces. They receive the bill two weeks later ($88). The occupational therapist recommends over-the-counter ankle supports for both ankles, which Marya finds very helpful in decreasing her pain ($50). Marya's wrist movements are increasingly painful, and the physiotherapist recommends regular warm wax treatments at home. The device for warm wax treatments costs $425. The family opts for a double boiler ($40) and buys the first batch of wax at the grocery store ($8); however, mom and dad worry about the safety of implementing the wax treatments at home.

The physician recommends methotrexate, an immune system suppressant. Neither of the parents has a drug plan through their employment. The drug costs $38/month, and Marya requires three refills before her next appointment ($114). Between appointments, the family has access to the city hospital's nurse clinician, who provides expertise via phone consultation as needed. Due to complications with medication, it has been necessary to consult the nurse clinician five times since Marya's last appointment ($70 long distance charges). Marya develops movement restricting deformities in some of her fingers. Her parents try to negotiate some adjustment with her school, and they are told that they will have to go through a process of having Marya declared disabled in order to obtain the laptop computer ($1,500) she needs to be able to write in class. Dad works with his extended family to navigate the application process, but Marya must go without the computer and is unable to take notes without a high level of pain, for at least her first term in grade 2. Marya's parents strongly desire the expertise of a naturopathic physician who will work with their rheumatologist ($125 initial consultation). They have friends who have had very encouraging results with such an arrangement, and there is a highly respected naturopath with a rural practice near their home. They cannot afford the naturopath.

Total Cost: $650
Rurality Tax/visit: $220 (return trip gas and mileage, phone charges between visits)
The Family's Minimum Annual Rurality Tax (10 visits): $2,800

Marya's situation is not dissimilar to the expenses and constraints experienced by thousands of Canadian families with children who have chronic conditions. Her story illustrates the myth of universality in Canadian health care access. Marya's long-term prognosis will undoubtedly be heavily influenced by her family's socioeconomic circumstances. Parental unemployment at any time in the course of Marya's illness will have a devastating effect on their ability to maintain contact with health services, and thus on Marya's health. Her family's rural location sets in motion an ongoing rurality tax, which is inconsistent with her legal right to health care. Rurality tax is defined as the extra amount of money that rural and remote individuals and families must pay if they are to have the same possibilities of access to health care as urban people. If Marya's family is from a racialized group, she will experience additional and powerful barriers related to racism in the health care system.

Source: Adapted from McGibbon 2009.

social determinants of health and the isms, what we have, ultimately, are intersections of intersections. Taken together, the intersecting areas — the SDH, the isms as SDH, and geography as SDH — create a powerful synergy of oppression that is very difficult to disentangle in terms of its policy base and its impact on everyday life. A clear example involves childhood asthma. As the discussion earlier in the chapter demonstrates, asthma outcomes in childhood are intimately tied to economic status related to social class, regardless of the child's individual biophysical and genetic characteristics. When families cannot afford relatively mould-free housing, children with asthma have more episodes of asthma and more admissions to the emergency department due to serious complications, if the family can even afford transportation to the service. Here we have intersections of many of the SDH all combining to strongly disadvantage poorer children: income and its inequitable distribution, housing insecurity and erosion of social safety nets. These intersections can also be readily demonstrated to include considerations about early childhood development, food insecurity and inaccessibility of health care services for poorer families (McGibbon, 2009).

Identity (the isms) and geography are also SDH. Thus, we can envision how complex and deeply embedded this system of disadvantage is for many children with asthma: if the child is from an Indigenous or Black family, or any family of colour, they will be dealing with well documented racism in the health care system. If they live in a rural area, access to specialist services will be seriously decreased (McGibbon, 2009). If they live in an area that has major motor vehicle traffic flow, as is often the case near low-income urban housing, they will have the added disadvantage of breathing toxic fuel emissions. Taken together, the SDH, identity as an SDH and geography as an SDH create a complex system of disadvantage that health and public policy is not yet equipped to tackle in Canada. Even the concept of intersectoral children's policy intervention has historically had difficulty gaining a foothold in public policy (McPherson, Popp, & Lindstrom, 2006). Box 2.1 provides a case example of how intersectionality unfolds in the everyday life of a Canadian family with a daughter who has juvenile rheumatoid arthritis.

Anchoring Change in the Structural Determinants of Health

The discussion and evidence presented in this chapter provide clear evidence of the inscription of oppression on mind, body, and spirit — the threats of oppression. These are the ways that the structural determinants of health are borne out in everyday life. Suffering and deprivation in individuals, families and communities is articulated to a complex network of economic and social policies over time. Chronic health problems, including those that lead to early death, are a result of inequitable health and social policies and the neoliberal ideology that underpins these policies. Engel's (2009 [1845]) treatise on social murder over a century and a half ago remains urgently relevant today. In order to address oppression in the area of the social determinants of health, it is crucial to take aim at the structural, policy-based causes of ill health and early death and thus create a socially relevant grounding for policy change for peoples under threat. The chapters in Part Three of this volume provide a detailed accounting of how these policy changes may come about.

3

Critical Perspectives on the Social Determinants of Health

Dennis Raphael

> One thing only is astounding, that class prejudice and preconceived opinions can hold a whole class of human beings in such perfect, I might almost say, such mad blindness. Meanwhile, the development of the nation goes its way whether the bourgeoisie has eyes for it or not, and will surprise the property-holding class one day with things not dreamed of in its philosophy. (Engels 2009 [1845]: 157)

The term "social determinants of health" (SDH) has achieved star status within Canadian health policy documents produced by the federal government (Public Health Agency of Canada, 2007, 2008), the Chief Health Officer of Canada (Butler-Jones, 2008) and the Canadian Senate (Senate Subcommittee on Population Health, 2008); numerous public health and social development organizations and agencies (Canadian Public Health Association, 2008; Chronic Disease Alliance of Ontario, 2008; White, Sterniczuk, Ramsay et al., 2006); research funding agencies (CIHR, 2005; Institute of Population and Public Health, 2003); and even the business-oriented Conference Board of Canada (2008). All concur that social determinants of health are the primary influences upon the health of individuals, communities and jurisdictions, whether health is defined medically as avoiding disease or more broadly as the extent to which Canadians are provided with the physical, social, and personal resources to identify and achieve personal aspirations, satisfy needs, and cope with the environment. All suggest that social determinants of health are about the quantity and quality of a variety of resources a society makes available to its members, implying that something should be done to strengthen them.

Despite the proliferation of documents concerning themselves with the SDH, actual implementation of these concepts in Canada lags well behind other jurisdictions (CPHI, 2002; Lavis, 2002; Raphael, Curry-Stevens, & Bryant, 2008). Much of this has to with the incompatibility of SDH concepts — and their public-policy implications — with current governmental approaches to issues of income and wealth distribution, program provision and state intervention in the operation of the dominant societal institutions in Canada and the marketplace (Raphael & Bryant, 2006). The result is the creation Canada's reputation as a "health promotion powerhouse," while the actual reality is one of increasing social and economic inequalities, deteriorating quality SDH and decaying health status and quality of life (Bryant, Raphael, Schrecker, et al., 2009)

In addition, due to a reticence among governmental and agency authorities to publicize these concepts too loudly, accompanied by a profound unwillingness on the part of the media to communicate these issues, public awareness and understanding of these concepts are, at best, minimal (CPHI, 2004b; Collins, Abelson, & Eyles, 2007; Eyles, Brimacombe, Chaulk, et al., 2001). The result is a disconnect between these SDH-related policy documents and actual public policymaking that is so profound as to suggest each is residing within parallel but non-interacting universes (Raphael, 2009b).

An additional problem is that even among SDH researchers and those attempting to implement SDH-related concepts, there is a reluctance to identify the public-policy implications of the SDH concept (Raphael, Macdonald, Labonte et al., 2004). There is an even greater reluctance to consider the political and ideological sources of the inequitable distribution of the quality of SDH among Canadians (Raphael, 2006). In this chapter I build upon Wright's (1994) concept of "economic oppression" to consider SDH-related oppression with regards to the SDH and their inequitable distribution among Canadians. For Wright, economic oppression is where "the material welfare of one group of people is causally related to the material deprivations of another" and "involves coercively enforced exclusion from access to productive resources" (2003: 376). The nature of this process is such that it is clearly "morally indictable." In the SDH adaptation, SDH-related oppression is the situation in which:

- individuals experiencing adverse-quality SDH do so because others experience excessively favourable SDH;
- individuals experiencing adverse quality SDH — low income; insecure employment, food and housing; lack of health and social services; and social exclusion — have no means of having policymakers address their situations; and
- these processes are clearly unjust and unfair.

By identifying the sources of SDH-related oppression — the governmental and institutional structures and processes as well as the groups and individuals that support these structures and processes — it becomes possible to find the means by which these pressures and forces can be altered. Failure to explicitly identify these sources will lead to further research, analysis, and document production on SDH that does little to shift the distribution of SDH in Canadian society. In the following sections I examine various ways of thinking about SDH, noting their contributions and deficiencies, and then outline means of advancing the SDH agenda.

Defining the Social Determinants of Health

SDH refer to the societal factors — and the unequal distribution of these factors — that contribute to both the overall health of Canadians and to existing inequalities in health (Graham, 2004). An SDH analysis contrasts with the usual preoccupation of governmental authorities, disease associations and the media with biomedical discoveries, health care advances and behavioural risk factors (Gasher, 2007; Hayes, Ross, Gasherc, et al., 2007; Legowski & McKay, 2000). Since the modern introduction of the term SDH (Tarlov, 1996), a variety of conceptualizations — all clearly referring to societal factors — have appeared (see Table 3.1).

Raphael et al.'s (2004) twelve social determinants of health, the last column in Table 3.1, are especially relevant to Canadians. These determinants are consistent with most existing formulations, understandable to the lay public and align with existing governmental structures and policy frameworks (e.g., Ministries of Education, Housing, Labour, Native Affairs, Women's Issues, etc.). *Social Determinants of Health: Canadian Perspectives* (Raphael, 2008b) provides an analysis of the current state of these determinants in Canada.

The evidence points to societal conditions, rather than biomedical and behavioural risk factors (the traditional focus), as the primary determinants of health (CSDH, 2008; Davey Smith, 2003; Wilkinson & Marmot, 2003). Since an SDH approach identifies the sources of health as being related to how a society organizes and distributes economic and social resources — a concept clearly implied in all the SDH conceptualizations provided in Table 3.1 — it should direct attention to economic and social policies as a means of improving the health of citizens. An SDH analysis should thus consider the political, economic and social forces that shape these policy decisions (Bambra, Fox, & Scott-Samuel, 2005).

Despite these conceptualizations and related empirical work, there has been little application of these concepts in the making of Canadian public policy. Since Canadians have little awareness of the important role that living conditions play in determining health, there is limited public pressure to have governments address the SDH. A main problem then is how to shift public knowledge to harness the powerful SDH message in the service of creating health-enhancing public policy. But what form should knowledge of the SDH take? Even among those conversant with the term, there are important differences in how the concept is understood and applied.

Table 3.1. Conceptualizations of the Social Determinants of Health

Ottawa Charter[1]	Dahlgren and Whitehead[2]	Health Canada[3]	World Health Organization[4]	Centres for Disease Control[5]	Raphael et at.[6]
peace	agriculture and food production	income and social status	social gradient	socio-economic status	Aboriginal status
shelter	education	social support networks	stress	transportation	early life
education	work environment	education	early life	housing	education
food	unemployment	employment and working conditions	social exclusion	access to services	employment and working conditions
income	water and sanitation	physical and social environments	work	discrimination by social grouping	food security
stable ecosystem	health care services	healthy child development	unemployment	social or environmental stressors	gender
sustainable resources	housing	health services	social support		health care services
social justice		gender	addiction		housing
equity		culture	food		income and its distribution
			transport		social safety net
					social exclusion
					unemployment and employment security

Sources: *1. World Health Organization, 1986; 2. Dahlgren & Whitehead, 1992; 3. Health Canada, 1998; 4. Wilkinson & Marmot, 2003; 5. Centers for Disease Control and Prevention, 2005; 6. Raphael, Bryant, & Curry-Stevens, 2004.*

Differing SDH Discourses

Within the health research and professional communities there is somewhat greater awareness of the SDH concept, and while there may even be a consensus that non-medical and non-behavioural risk factors are worthy of attention, profound differences exist in how this consensus plays out in research and professional activity. This is not merely about differing paradigms, which define intellectual world views about phenomena and how such phenomena can be understood or investigated (Guba, 1990; Kuhn, 1970). They actually represent *discourses,* which — as defined by Michael Foucault — exert a much more powerful influence. According to Lessa (2006: 285):

> Foucault (1972) refers to discourses as systems of thoughts composed of ideas, attitudes, courses of actions, beliefs and practices that systematically construct the subjects and the worlds of which they speak. He traces the role of discourses in wider social processes of legitimating and power, emphasizing the constitution of current truths, how they are maintained and what power relations they carry with them.

Differing SDH discourses assume great importance as their varying parameters have the power to direct the kinds of research and professional activities that are deemed acceptable, that is, fundable in the case of research applications and institutional budgeting and career-enhancing, that is, not espousing a view that is "out of bounds" so that one's future prospects are not hampered. Different SDH discourses can thus have the following different effects:

- limit focus, analysis and action to medical, behavioural and health care issues, thereby neglecting how SDH-generated social and material deprivation shape health;
- consider how SDH affect health but neglect how SDH come to be unequally distributed as a result of public-policy decisions;
- identify specific groups that experience poor quality SDH but fail to place these findings within a broader public-policy context;
- examine public-policy aspects of SDH but neglect the economic, political and ideological forces that shape how public policy is made; and
- point out how societal structures shape the SDH and their distribution, but fail to specify how specific classes and groups both create and benefit from the inequitable distribution of the SDH, and identify means by which their influence can be countered.

Related to these issues is whether an SDH discourse limits activity to research and analysis, thereby avoiding commitments to action, bringing to mind Marx's famous dictum: "The philosophers have only interpreted the world in various ways. The point however, is to change it." In the following sections I examine the contribution — and deficiencies — of the discourses summarized in Table 3.1 and how they play out in terms of Canadian research activity and professional practice.

Discourse 1: SDH as Identifiers of Canadians Requiring Specific Health and Social Services

The health care and social services communities recognize that individuals and communities experiencing adverse SDH have a greater incidence of a variety of medical problems. For them, SDH represent a set of adverse living conditions that should direct the targeting of various services to vulnerable individuals. Significant effort is expended in identifying the health and social service needs of individuals who experience adverse SDH. Specific areas of concern have included health care needs of homeless individuals, management of chronic diseases of vulnerable communities, and promoting screening and primary health care among immigrant groups, among others (Benoit, Carroll, & Chaudhry, 2003; Hwang & Bugeja, 2000; Saxena, Majeed, & Jones, 1999; Sword, 2000). Public health focuses on providing preventive and supportive services to various socioeconomic and ethnic groups. Social service agencies strive to reach out and support individuals experiencing adverse living situations.

The provision of responsive and sensitive health and social services are important. But limiting activity to developing and implementing such programs and neglecting the sources of material and social deprivation — i.e., poor quality SDH — that create health and social problems will do little to reduce the needs for these services. Community health centres across Canada are somewhat unique in implementing this discourse, but *also* striving to educate clients, governmental authorities, and the general public as to the importance of improving the SDH that are the sources of adverse health (Albrecht, 1998; Association of Ontario Health Centres, 2007). However, without such broader activity, this discourse has the potential to reinforce the already dominant health care and social service emphases, thereby continuing to obscure the importance to health of the SDH and their inequitable distribution.

Discourse 2: SDH as Identifiers of Canadians with Modifiable Medical and Behavioural Risk Profiles

Similarly, those concerned with promoting "healthy lifestyles" recognize that individuals and communities experiencing adverse SDH are more likely to exhibit a whole range of medical (e.g., high blood sugar and "bad" cholesterol levels) and behavioural (e.g., poor diet, lack of physical activity, tobacco and excessive alcohol use) risk factors. For them, the SDH represent a set of adverse living conditions that direct attention to modifying risk behaviours among those experiencing adverse SDH (Allison, Adlaf, Ialomiteanu, et al., 1999; Choi & Shi, 2001; Choiniere, Lafontaine, & Edwards, 2000; Potvin, Richard, & Edwards, 2000).

Unlike Discourse 1, which identifies the need to provide clearly important health and social services to Canadians experiencing poor quality SDH, this discourse and its implementation have significant negative aspects. First, the medical and behavioural risk factors account for relatively little of the variation in health outcomes when compared to the experience of poor quality SDH (Lantz, House, Lepkowski, et al., 1998; Raphael, Anstice, & Raine, 2003; Raphael & Farrell, 2002). Second, the discourse is embedded within a framework that assumes that individuals are capable of "making healthy lifestyle choices," such that those who fail to do so are seen as responsible for their own adverse health outcomes (Labonte & Penfold, 1981; Raphael, 2002). Third, evidence indicates that these programs demonstrate rather little effectiveness, serving only to further disenable vulnerable populations and the "healthy lifestyle" agencies and workers administering these programs (O'Loughlin, 2001; Raphael, 2002). Finally, this discourse has a disturbing tendency to neglect the sources of the adverse SDH to which Canadians are exposed, further obscuring their importance (Raphael, 2003). Despite these clear deficiencies, this discourse dominates most government and local public health activity and is the mainstay of disease-association communication. Reinforced by the media, it reinforces the "lifestyle" understandings of the Canadian public as to the sources of health and makes communication of even the basic SDH message difficult if not impossible.

Discourse 3: SDH as Indicators of
Material Living Conditions That Shape Health

In this discourse there is clear recognition that adverse SDH themselves are important influences upon health and that various pathways exist by which adverse quality SDH "get under the skin" to shape health. One influential model identifies interacting material, psychological and behavioural pathways that are influenced by social structures (broadly defined), employment and working conditions, and neighbourhood characteristics (Brunner & Marmot, 2006). Other models specify how exposures to poor quality SDH during childhood and adulthood interact to produce health outcomes across the lifespan (Benzeval, Dilnot, Judge, et al. , 2001; van de Mheen, Stronks, & Mackenbach, 1998). Models identifying physiological processes by which the SDH "get under the skin" are another area of activity (Brunner & Marmot, 2006; Meany, Szyf, & Seckl, 2007; Sapolsky, 1992).

The specification of latent, pathway and cumulative exposures during childhood as shaping health across the lifespan has also directed attention to the importance of the SDH (Hertzman, 1994, 1999). There is extensive evidence of the importance for health of each SDH domain (e.g., Aboriginal status, early life, education, employment and working conditions, food security, gender, health care services, housing, income and its distribution, social safety net, social exclusion, and unemployment and employment security) (see Raphael, 2008b). The clear message of this discourse is that the material, psychological and behavioural effects of adverse living conditions — not the adoption of poor "lifestyle" choices — are the primary determinants of health.

Yet even this more mature SDH discourse can be diluted if the public-policy antecedents of SDH are not emphasized. Governments and health and social service organizations and agencies may take information about the importance of early life, for instance, and translate this into being about parents' behaviours toward their children. They then focus upon promoting better parenting or fostering more physical exercise in schools rather than improving the SDH by increasing financial resources or providing affordable housing. Authorities may implement breakfast programs, clothing and food drives, and coping or anger-management classes rather than consider how public policies create financial insecurity. Specifying public policy antecedents of SDH and their distribution would seem essential to any SDH agenda.

Discourse 4: SDH as Indicators of Material Living Circumstances That Differ as a Function of Group Membership

There is also an active literature concerned with variations in the SDH and health status of Canadians that occur as a function of class, gender, and race (Dunn & Dyck, 2000; Galabuzi, 2004; McMullin, 2008; Ornstein, 2000; Pederson & Raphael, 2006; Wallis & Kwok, 2008). This work draws upon the extensive social inequalities literature and specifies how particular groups are exposed to poor quality SDH. This important work identifies how particular groups are vulnerable to health-threatening living conditions. It has the potential to mobilize Canadians to address these differences. But like the previous discourse, this work lends itself to the possibility — if the public-policy antecedents of the inequitable distribution of SDH are not emphasized — of seeing the problem as being amenable to program interventions (e.g., literacy and counselling programs, anti-discrimination training, etc.) directed towards individuals or groups.

Discourse 5: SDH and Their Distribution as Results of Public-policy Decisions Made by Governments and Other Societal Institutions

> This unequal distribution of health-damaging experiences is not in any sense a "natural" phenomenon but is the result of a toxic combination of poor social policies and programmes, unfair economic arrangements, and bad politics. (CSDH, 2008, p. 1)

As noted, SDH discourse can identify the relationship between a social determinant of health and health status such as lower income, food insecurity or inadequate housing, and show how it is related to poor health. In this discourse the analysis is extended to consider how SDH and their distribution come about as a result of public-policy decisions. As a result there is a clear assumption that the primary means of improving the SDH and promoting their more equitable distribution is through action to promote SDH-supporting public policy. This discourse is well represented by the conclusions of the World Health Organization's Commission on the Social Determinants of Health (2008).

As an illustration of this discourse, the SDH of early life is shaped by availability of material resources that assure adequate educational opportunities, food and housing, among other SDH (Hertzman, 2000). Much of this has to do with parents' employment security, wages, and the quality of their working conditions (Innocenti Research Centre, 2007). The availability of quality, regulated childcare is an especially important policy option in support of early life (Esping-Andersen, 2002). All of these SDH are shaped by public policy. Table 3.2 provides a summary of SDH public-policy antecedents.

Despite this recognition, there is a striking unwillingness among many SDH researchers and workers to explicitly outline the public-policy antecedents of SDH and their distribution (Raphael, 2008b). Kirkpatrick comments on this tendency in regards to the Chief Public Health Officer of Canada's (CPHO) recent report on health inequalities in Canada:

> The CPHO report's failure to emphasize the essential role of government action is reinforced by the examples used to illustrate "successful interventions that... may serve to reduce Canada's health inequalities and improve quality of life for all Canadians" (p. 1). In fact, the interventions highlighted tend to be community-based programs that are unable to address the structural determinants of health inequalities. (Kirkpatrick & McIntyre, 2009 p. 94)

It is unclear why this is the case. It may be that SDH researchers and workers trained within the assumptions of so-called "objective" science are sensitive to the accusation that such analyses are "political." It is more likely that there is a perception that such analyses — likely as they are to be critical of current government public-policy approaches — may threaten research and program funding, weaken regard by professional colleagues and ultimately threaten career prospects. The profound lack of training in public-policy analysis by most health-related researchers and workers also cannot be disregarded.

Table 3.2: SDH and Their Public-Policy Antecedents

Determinants	Public-Policy Antecedents
Aboriginal status	culturally appropriate education, social and health care services, control over local community institutions
early life	adequate income either inside or outside of the work force, availability of quality childcare and early education, support services
education	support for literacy initiatives, greater public spending, tuition policy
employment and working conditions	training and retraining programs (active labour policy), support for union organizing and collective bargaining, increasing worker input into workplaces
food security	developing adequate income and poverty-reduction policies, promoting healthy food policy, providing affordable housing
gender	pay equity legislation, access to employment benefits, affordable and quality childcare
health services	managing resources effectively, providing comprehensive accessible, responsive and timely care
housing	providing adequate income and affordable housing, reasonable rental controls and housing supplements, providing social housing for those in need
income and income distribution	equitable taxation policy, adequate minimum wages, social assistance levels that support health
social exclusion	developing and enforcing anti-discrimination laws, providing ESL and job training, approving foreign credentials, supporting a variety of other health determinants
social safety net	providing social assistance, unemployment and retraining supports comparable to those provided in other developed nations
unemployment and employment security	active labour policy, providing adequate replacement benefits, labour laws that promote job security

Discourse 6: SDH and Their Distribution as Results of
Economic and Political Structures and Justifying Ideologies

> Our analysis makes an empirical link between politics and policy,
> by showing that political parties with egalitarian ideologies tend
> to implement redistributive policies. An important finding of our
> research is that policies aimed at reducing social inequalities, such as
> welfare state and labour market policies, do seem to have a salutary
> effect on the selected health indicators, infant mortality and life ex-
> pectancy at birth. (Navarro, Muntaner, Benach, et al., 2006: abstract)

Identifying public-policy antecedents of SDH and their distribution can promote and support public-policy advocacy. Such activity is consistent with
models that see policymaking as a rational exercise by which government
authorities listen to citizens, calculate benefits and costs, and then make
decisions (Brooks & Miljan, 2003a). The problem with this analysis is that it
doesn't seem to account for how SDH-related public policy is made in Canada.

Why is it that many nations have acted upon SDH-related evidence, while
Canada is identified as an SDH policy laggard (Bryant, Raphael, Schrecker,
et al., 2009)? In Discourse 6 the analysis is on how Canada's and other nations' historical traditions and economic and political structures support
or hinder SDH-supportive public policies. Jurisdictional approaches to SDH
issues cluster such that they can be said to represent entirely different welfare
state regimes (Raphael & Bryant, 2006). The "worlds of welfare" analysis
identifies three distinct types of welfare states that illuminate these issues
(Bambra, 2007; Eikemo & Bambra, 2008): social democratic (e.g., Sweden,
Norway, Denmark, Finland), liberal (e.g., U.S., U.K., Canada, Ireland)
and conservative (e.g., France, Germany, Netherlands, Belgium) (Esping-
Andersen, 1990, 1999).

Figure 3.1 is a graphic interpretation by two Canadian sociologists of
how differences in political and economic structures and processes (political
economy) — themselves a result of historical traditions and governance by
specific political parties over time — are related to the SDH (Saint-Arnaud &
Bernard, 2003). In addition, scholarship demonstrates that the social democratic welfare states provide far superior quality SDH (e.g., equitable income
distribution and low poverty rates; family supports including early education
and care, living wages; progressive employment policies; food and housing
security; extensive health and social services, etc.) — than liberal welfare states
(Conference Board of Canada, 2003, 2006; Innocenti Research Centre, 2008;
Navarro, Muntaner, Benach, et al., 2006; Navarro & Shi, 2002; OECD, 2009;
Raphael, 2007a). Not surprisingly, on numerous health and quality-of-life
indicators, the social democratic political economies outperform the liberal
(Conference Board of Canada, 2003, 2006; Navarro et al., 2004). Chapter 12

Figure 3.1: Ideological Variations in Forms of the Welfare State

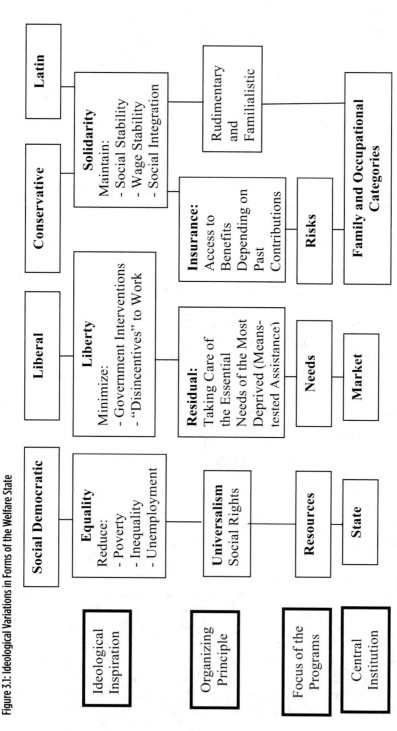

Source: *Saint-Arnaud and Bernard, 2003:. 503.*

of this volume provides further discussion of a political economy perspective in understanding and ameliorating the paths to oppression that cause inequities in health and well-being.

Since the dominant inspiration of liberal political economies is to minimize government intervention in the operation of its central institution — the market — it should not be surprising that Canada, and its liberal partners, fall well behind other nations in addressing the unequal distribution of the SDH. It should also not be surprising that Canadian public policy continues to be adverse to SDH concepts. How then does one go about promoting public policy within liberal political economies?

Discourse 7: SDH and Their Distribution as Results of the Power/Influence of Those Who Create and Benefit from Social and Health Inequalities

> It is not inequalities that kill, but those who benefit from the inequalities that kill. (Navarro, 2009, p. 15)

This final discourse identifies the individuals and groups in Canada who, through their undue influence upon governments, create and benefit from social and health inequalities, and in the process weaken the SDH and skew their distribution. These individuals and groups have successfully lobbied for shifting the tax structures to favour the corporate sector and the wealthy, reducing public expenditures, controlling wages and employment benefits, and relaxing labour standards and protections (Chernomas & Hudson, 2009; Langille, 2008; McBride & Shields, 1997; McQuaig, 1987, 1993; Scarth, 2004). These public-policy changes have led to striking increases in income and wealth among the already wealthy in Canada and also to increasing income and wealth inequalities, stagnating incomes for most Canadians and increased housing and food insecurity (Jackson, 2000; Kerstetter, 2002; Lee, 2007). As a result, Canada has come to have one of the most undeveloped welfare states — with attendant weak SDH-related public policy — among the wealthy developed nations (Raphael, 2007a).

Who exactly are these villains and how can their undue influence upon public policy be resisted? Consistent with analyses that the marketplace is the dominant institution in Canada, Langille (2008) identifies business associations such as the Canadian Bankers Association and the Canadian Chamber of Commerce; think tanks such as the C.D. Howe Institute and the Fraser Institute; citizen-front institutions such as the Canadian Taxpayers Federation and the National Citizens Coalition, and lobbyists such as Earnscliffe and Hill and Knowlton, as important advocates for SDH-weakening public policy. Chernomas and Hudson (2009: 120) argue:

The gulf between the promises of conservative economic policy and its results is becoming increasingly clear. While conservative economic policy promises economic benefits for the vast majority of the population, in reality, income, power, and privilege have been shifted toward those who own and control the corporate world and away from the majority of the North American population. The current conservative policy environment has made our society less healthy, more dangerous, less stable, more unequal, less fair, and more inefficient.

It is important to recognize that these individuals and groups are acting in their own interests, and in a parliamentary democracy they have every right to do so. The problem is that, as their power and influence have increased, there have been corresponding declining counterbalances to their influence (Langille, 2008; McBride & Shields, 1997). What form might these counterbalances take? Langille (2008) and others propose educating the public and using strength in numbers to promote public policy that will oppose this agenda.

Wright's (1994, 2003) argument for organizing to "oppose and defeat" the powerful interests that influence governments to maintain poverty can be applied to support the equitable distribution of the SDH. These defeats can occur in the workplace through greater union organization and increasing public recognition of the class-related forces that shape public policy. Defeats can also occur in the electoral and parliamentary arena by election of political parties that favour public-policy action to strengthen the SDH (Brady, 2003; Esping-Andersen, 1985). Internationally, it is well demonstrated that social democratic political parties are more receptive to — and successful at — implementing SDH-supportive public policies (Brady, 2003; Navarro, 2009; Rainwater & Smeeding, 2003). In Canada, the NDP — in contrast to the Liberal and Conservative Parties — have policy positions more consistent with enhancing the SDH. (Raphael, 2007b). Navarro and Shi argue:

> For those wishing to optimize the health of populations by reducing social and income inequalities, it seems advisable to support political forces such as the labor movement and social democratic parties which have traditionally supported larger, more distributive policies than have the Christian democratic or liberal parties. (Navarro & Shi, 2001, p. 20)

These parties could work to restore social programs and services and reintroduce more progressive income tax rates. Parties of the left have more influence under electoral systems that apply proportional representation (PR), and PR has been on the Canadian public-policy agenda for years (Alesina & Glaeser, 2004; Esping-Andersen, 1985).

Outside of the electoral process, making it easier to organize unions and re-regulating many industries would provide a counterbalance to the increasing concentration of influence and wealth of the corporate and business sectors (Zweig, 2000). The provision of a social wage — government provided services that people need to live and develop their ability to work — and restoring the social infrastructure that has been so weakened in nations such as Canada would also strengthen the SDH and provide more equitable distribution of these resources. Resistance to the privatization of public services, which tends to weaken SDH, is also essential (Zweig, 2004).

Conclusion

Efforts to strengthen the SDH through public-policy activity in Canada lag well behind those in other developed nations. Government authorities are resistant to the SDH concept, and public lack of awareness minimizes the likelihood of public pressure to address these issues. Even within the SDH research and professional community there is resistance to exploring the public-policy implications of the unequal distribution of SDH. Various discourses that consider the SDH but ignore their public-policy antecedents allow government authorities to neglect the SDH and their inequitable distribution.

The most mature discourse — and one that clearly recognizes the role that oppression plays in SDH and their inequitable distribution — proposes addressing these issues through public-policy action in the political realm. Achieving this action will require educating the public that deteriorating quality SDH and inequitable SDH distribution result from the undue influence upon public policymaking by those creating and profiting from social and health inequalities. In light of Canada's current economic and political structures and the continuing influence of the corporate and business sector upon public policymaking, the possibility of achieving significant progress on SDH-related issues by working within the other discourses seems unlikely.

Part 2

How Oppression Operates
to Produce Health Inequities

Fragmented Performances

Ageism and the Health of Older Women

Raewyn Bassett

"Aging" has become a euphemism for "old age." The focus on life stages (e.g., adolescence) and age cohorts (e.g., boomers) assumes homogeneity between those so categorized and pits one life stage and cohort against another. Each, of course, is closely aligned with a specific range of ages. The age category "sixty-five years and over" is used in the literature to denote "old age," although many women observe that there are other signifiers of age used to define them before they ever reach sixty-five, for example greying hair and "crow's feet."

"Old age" is a diffuse category at one end of a continuum that begins at birth, its boundaries leaking out of and into "middle age." At the other end of the continuum it heads in a single direction to an uncontrollable fate (Gullette, 2004). Locating a term that situates and defines older women respectfully, yet is not replete with ageist ideology, is next to impossible. A search of the Oxford Online Dictionary provided terms such as "elder: of a greater age; older: having lived for a long time, no longer young; senior: of or relating to a more advanced age," all of which are used often in the literature and to which varying ages are attached. Indeed, all women are elder, older and senior when compared to the age cohort previous to them. "Elder" is often invoked as more respectful than other terms because of its implicit reference to wisdom; however, wisdom as a social role for older women, based on their knowledge and experience accumulated over a long period of time, is dismissed or ignored in Western societies (Woodward, 2002). I primarily use the term "older" in this chapter to designate this diffuse category of women perceived as "old" and "aging."

Accompanying the term "aging" is a narrative of decline that is related exclusively to the physical body designated as "old" (Overall, 2006; Gullette, 2004). Yet it is not our declining bodies that age us so much as cultural and social structures. As "beings who age" (Gullette, 2004, p. 112) we are influenced by social factors such as poverty, racism, sexism, ageism and environmental degradation, among others. Good health begins in the first years of life, even before birth (Dillaway & Byrnes, 2009; Gullette, 2004). The inequalities that show themselves on and in the bodies of women in later life have accumulated over a lifetime (Ferraro & Shippee, 2009). Age theorists take for granted that social disadvantage overlays a biologically given old age but do not recognize that biologically given old age as socially constructed. There is no given number of years that constitute old age, only the years that are selected and defined as "old". At any time, "aging" can be redefined, by expanding or retracting the chronological age that represents the old age category (Overall, 2006).

In this chapter, I begin with the narrative that emerges from Health Canada's statistics regarding health outcomes for women aged sixty-five years and over. I then turn to the discourses of aging in an attempt to understand this narrative of the health of older women. These discourses place responsibility for decline and disability associated with aging firmly with older women. Finally, I elaborate the ageist assumptions contained within aging discourses, together with how they influence the care women provide for themselves and that is provided to them by their health professionals. These ageist discourses are subtle, often tacit, forms of oppression that impact women's lives. They are the stories we tell ourselves and that are told to us in the media, by our families, by health professionals and others and that frame how we and others recognize us. They are regimes of truth (Foucault, 1980) that designate who and what will, and will not, be recognized (Butler, 2001). That is, the discourses offer a framework that delineates who qualifies as a subject and provides the norms by which the subject will be recognized. The performance of aging, however, is not to be taken for granted; it is not set in stone. On the contrary, it is a fragmented performance as women move between recognizing themselves through the discourses of aging and understanding themselves outside these discourses.

The Health of Women Aged Sixty-Five and Over

Many Canadian women are living longer (Shields & Martel, 2005) and are healthier than previous generations (Rotermann, 2005). Despite this improvement in life expectancy and well-being, the picture painted by health statistics portrays growing older as a process of decline. Comparison with Canadians below the age of sixty-five years shows that older people suffer more from chronic conditions, are inactive and require assistance in daily activities (Shields & Chen, 1999). Of those Canadians over the age of sixty-five, women are worse off than men. On the one hand, 52 percent of women over the age of sixty-five in 2003 were described as having overall good health, including good functional health, independent activities of daily living and good to excellent self-perceived mental and general health. On the other hand, when compared with men sixty-five and over, women were significantly lower in their ability to carry out independent activities of daily living and in functional health areas such as vision, hearing, mobility and freedom from pain (Shields & Martel, 2005).

Eighty-five percent of women aged sixty-five and over have at least one chronic condition (Statistics Canada, 2006a). In the two decades between 1978/79 and 1998/99, the prevalence of diabetes and asthma increased significantly among women sixty-five and older. Prevalence of arthritis, rheumatism, high blood pressure and migraine headaches is significantly higher among women than men in this age group (Shields & Chen, 1999). Women were significantly more likely than men to consult a family doctor, an eye specialist, a chiropractor, physiotherapist, alternative health care provider and social worker or counsellor. Illness, chronic conditions, injuries and fair to poor self-perceived health were the predominant determinants of visits to doctors and for hospitalization (Rotermann, 2005).

In 2002, the three leading causes of death for women over the age of sixty-five were heart disease (26 percent), cancer (24 percent) and Alzheimer's disease and stroke (9.3 percent). Women's risk of dying is strongly influenced by psychological distress and lack of adequate financial means to purchase necessities. Other factors include being widowed, inactive, underweight or functionally impaired; currently smoking or having quit for less than ten years; and suffering from stroke, diabetes or respiratory diseases (Wilkins, 2005).

In 2003, women over the age of sixty-five were reported as taking a wider variety of medicines and as having a higher likelihood of medication use than men of the same age. At the same time, women sixty-five and older were significantly less likely than men to use heart medication (F=19.8 percent; M=25.1 percent) and drugs for diabetes (F=7.7 percent; M=11.0 percent) (Rotermann, 2005) despite a greater mortality for women (24,064 in 2002) than men (21,950) in that age group from heart disease (Wilkins, 2005). In 2003, women sixty-five years and over were more likely than men to receive home care. Women are more likely to live alone, and these living arrangements, along with the need for help with activities of daily living, were the predominant factors in their increased need for home care. Chronic conditions, such as an activity-limiting injury, and fair to poor perceived health, also influence their need for home care (Rotermann, 2005).

Depression is the leading cause of disability among women (Gilmour, 2008); however, prevalence is lowest among the sixty-five and over age group (Statistics Canada, 1999). Older women reporting a strong sense of community belonging also reported good physical and mental health (72 percent of men and women aged sixty-five or older compared to 55 percent in eighteen to twenty-nine year olds, and 77 percent in adolescents twelve to seventeen years) (Shields, 2008). In a study of older women at senior centres in Montreal, high-quality dyadic relationships (among married, widowed, divorced, single with partners or remarried) positively and significantly affected overall feelings and happiness, suggesting that negative mental health feelings may be mediated by the quality of dyadic relationships (Fitzpatrick, 2009).

Late-life depression has been found to be associated with mild cognitive impairment (MCI) and dementia (Bhalla, Butters, Becker, et al., 2009). Half a million Canadians have Alzheimer's disease or a related dementia with 71,000 of them under age 65. Women represent 72 per cent of all Alzheimer's disease cases (Alzheimers Society of Canada, 2009). Alzheimer's disease is more predominant in women, and the prevalence of dementia increases sharply as women age beyond sixty-five years. Women with dementia, more so than men, are cared for in institutions and for longer periods of time, mainly because of the absence of a spouse or family-member caregiver (Hill, Forbes, Berthelot, et al., 1996).

Canadian data show that as women age the risk of domestic violence declines (Statistics Canada, 2005a), suggesting they may outlive their abusers or that their partners are no longer physically capable of abuse. At the same time, statistics show that 30 percent of male perpetrators of violence against older women were men aged sixty-fvie and over, suggesting that spousal violence cannot be discounted. In 2007, one-third of family violence incidents reported to police were committed against older adults. A family member, for example, a current or former spouse or an adult child, was the most common perpetrator of violence against senior women. Physical injury was seldom the result, and when it did occur, was minor (Statistics Canada, 2009). Few older women used shelters in response to abuse. In 2008, 180 women fifty-five years and over were residing in shelters for reasons of abuse on the day the survey snapshot of women's shelter statistics was collected (Sauvé & Burns, 2009). Family violence was highest among seniors aged sixty-fvie to seventy-four and lowest among seniors eighty-five and older (Statistics Canada, 2009). Women over the age of sevety-four are more likely to live alone or in institutions, which may alleviate the abusive situation (Turcotte & Schellenberg, 2007). Health-related reasons (e.g., dementia) or social isolation resulting in the need to depend on family may also diminish reporting of violence by older women (Statistics Canada, 2009).

Homicide rates are low for older women (Statistics Canada, 2009). Of thirty-eight homicides in 2007 against seniors, sixteen were women. As in other forms of family violence, homicides of older women were most often committed by a spouse or adult son. Police-reported data on violence against seniors, however, underestimate the prevalence of these crimes. Seniors may not report violence against them, and police records do not capture other forms of violence, such as financial or psychological abuse and neglect (Statistics Canada, 2009). In addition, smaller qualitative studies in Canada suggest that violence occurs across generations: past child abuse, such abuse by parents or abuse residential schools may lead to elder abuse (Walsh, Ploeg, Lohfield, et al., 2007).

Concerns about the quality of life experienced by older Canadians are increasingly raised in the language of chronic conditions, functional decline and reduced perceptions about health. At the same time, the message received about aging is that poor health in advanced years is not inevitable and that risk factors can be modified to extend years lived in good health and to prolong life. In order to understand the decline narrative painted by the statistics about older Canadian women and the message that decline is not inevitable, I turn to the discourses about aging to explain conceptions about old age in Canadian society.

Discourses about Aging

Discourses refer to speech or writing, words or utterances which are embedded in, determined by and contribute to social contexts. Discourses frame the way we think about things by both excluding and including information. Embedded with values and beliefs (Mills, 1997), discourses have a reciprocal relationship with social, political and economic events (Herman, 2004). Although these discourses on aging had their beginnings in the 1960s when Havighurst (1961) suggested that successful aging include quality as well as quantity in years, it is in the unfolding of events at the turn of the century that healthy and successful aging have become the taken-for-granted, insidious narratives we now tell ourselves.

Normal aging is a process in which the intrinsic changes that accompany getting older increase the risk of disease and disability. Considered a natural process of growing older, a normal aging discourse legitimizes ill-health in old age (Jolanki, 2004). According to this discourse, physical decline inevitably results in a decrease in physical activity, disengagement from previous roles and activities and acceptance by older people of fundamental changes to their lifestyles (Wray, 2003). Until very recently, mandatory retirement heralded the arrival of old age for most individuals and was considered a well-deserved respite for many from a busy life of raising a family and contributing towards the national economy. Retirement was a just reward for the middle class for their contribution. The expectation was of aging "normally," where decline was inevitable but not immediate. If you could afford to retire, the sunset of one's life was a time to relax, enjoy being older and forget about being regulated by work-day hours and rules. Responsibility for old age was shared between the state and the individual.

Today, the number of women and men who have arrived at "old age" has led to concern about how society can afford to meet the needs of this growing population bubble. A perceived apocalyptic demography whereby extended life expectancy no longer heralds progress, but instead presages an economic problem of "too many people living too long" (Asquith, 2009, p. 256) has required new discourses of healthy and successful aging, collectively termed *positive* aging. Developed in the United States by Butler (1990) and Rowe (1990) at a time when government was concerned about the burden of an aging population, productive and successful aging discourses added to the negative conceptualizations of old people. The then-current image of older people as unable to work (deserving poor) changed to an image of old people who were unwilling to work (undeserving poor), thus refocusing the perspective of older people's needs (Dillaway & Byrne, 2009).

To deter disease and disability, risky behaviours had to be avoided and strong physical health maintained (Rowe & Kahn, 1987). The absence of chronic illness and physical and functional limitations and perceived health as good to excellent was defined as healthy aging. The addition of physical activity and social connectedness recast healthy aging as successful aging (Asquith, 2009; Rowe & Kahn, 1987). Disease and disability are absent, cognitive and physical function and social interaction are maintained, and productive activities are pursued. Yet many women in later life who experience disease and disability age successfully, and conversely, many who are healthy may not age successfully as defined by these discourses (Sarkisian, Hays, & Mangione, 2002).

The ability to adapt physically and attitudinally to age limitations (von Faber, Bootsma-van der Wiel, van Exel, et al., 2001), to manage disability and disease, to remain socially engaged (Jang, Mortimer, Haley, et al., 2004) and to anticipate future events and the possibility of the unexpected, as well as to learn from past experiences (Fisher & Specht, 1999) were considered more important than the absence of disease and disability. Resiliency conferred by internal coping strategies and mental adjustments (Brandtstadter & Greve, 1994) buffers the effects of negative events (Smith, Borchelt, Maier, et al., 2002), including stereotypes of old age (Wray, 2003). Adaptation to growing old is further assisted by internal mechanisms of selection, compensation and optimization (Baltes & Carstensen, 1996), which contribute to an elder's positive interactions with others, sense of purpose, autonomy, personal growth, acceptance and environmental fit (Ryff, 1989).

Yet underlying these discourses of healthy, successful and positive aging is the medicalization of aging; its treatment individualized to prevent disease and disability (Clarke & Griffin, 2008) and "to combat deterioration and decay" (Featherston, Hepworth, & Turner, 1991, p. 170). There is also a moral imperative to arrive at old age disease- and disability-free and to maintain this healthy status throughout old age (Clarke & Griffin, 2008), thus curtailing the burden of welfare risk (Angus & Reeve, 2006). Successful aging is the responsibility of the individual, whose past lifestyle choices are evident in how she arrives at old age — chronically ill, disabled or healthy (Overall, 2006). However, these discourses do not recognize the multiplicity and flexibility of life trajectories and paths to successful aging (Ferraro & Shippee, 2009;

Scheidt, Humpherys, & Yorgason, 1999). Alternative perspectives on aging have been eclipsed by a myopic emphasis on coping with loss (Carstensen & Freund, 1994). Dominant assumptions about the meaning and attainment of contentment and happiness in later life infuse the successful aging discourses. The agency of older women is absent, and Western society's obsession with youth is reinforced (Wray, 2003). These discourses imply that individuals have control over their well-being, risk factors, mental health, engagement with others and whether they will contract disease (Dillaway & Byrnes, 2009).

More so than the focus on individuals, the positive and successful aging discourses fail to recognize that an aging population is a structural problem, generated in part by the economic needs of Western nation states in past decades (Asquith, 2009; Rottier & Jackson, 2003). Inequalities, in both risk and opportunity, are generated by social systems and accumulate over a lifetime (Ferraro & Shippee, 2009). Optimizing good health in old age begins in the first years of an individual's life, not in the last years, and requires not only individual responsibility but government support and appropriate cultural representations of aging (Dillaway & Byrnes, 2009; Calasanti, Slevin, & King, 2006; Gullette, 2004). Further, other inequalities intersect with old age. For example, the pursuit of an active "lifestyle" to stay fit is not available to older women who lack material and financial resources (Calasanti, Slevin & King, 2006). Health is causally related to socioeconomic status, particularly income and education (Buckley, Denton, Robb, et al, 2004), which in turn influences use of health services. More than 20 percent of older Canadian women have not engaged in paid labour and receive little or no employment pension benefits. Almost 25 percent of older women live below the poverty line (Spitzer, 2005). The current positive aging discourse is a misnomer, because it requires that people live long and do not show visible signs of aging, which is an impossibility (Featherson & Hepworth, 1995). If women cannot meet the benchmarks for aging successfully, then they are said to have failed — they have negatively aged (Asquith, 2009).

Ageism

Infused in the discourses on aging is ageism, an oppressive, hierarchical system of social relations based on age (Calasanti, 2007; Laws, 1995). Societies differentiate between age-related life stages and assign responsibilities and behaviours to each life stage (Calasanti, 2007). These intersect with the predominant value system in Western society, where individual status and value are located in economic productivity, performance and independence. Privilege and power, assigned on the basis of these and other values and status, accrue to life stages in relation to one another, shaping unequal interactions in ways that have material consequences. Some age groups benefit at the expense of others. For example, younger age groups face less competition for scarce resources such as work and income when compared to those in old age. By stigmatizing the oppressed group (older people), the privileged group (younger people) takes resources as a natural entitlement that might otherwise go to the oppressed group (Calasanti, 2007). The naturalization of entitlement of one group over another creates and maintains prejudices in which the characterization of age categories is exaggerated and homogenized into stereotypes, with the result that all people in later life are seen negatively (Angus & Reeve, 2006; Macionis & Gerber, 2005).

Stereotypes lead to prejudicial views held within society (Macionis & Gerber, 2005). They assist people to make sense of, and simplify, the complexities of everyday life, legitimizing and perpetuating discriminatory beliefs, attitudes and behaviours while simultaneously limiting others (Angus & Reeve, 2006). Difficult to change because they are often emotionally charged, stereotypes distort reality and unfairly blame individuals with little power for their perceived lack (Macionis & Gerber, 2005). Stereotypes based on age and ageist attitudes become embedded in institutions such as work, family and the health care system (Sharpe, 1995). Individual and systemic discrimination and prejudice influence scientific research, policies, programs and legislation regarding women in later life (Angus & Reeve, 2006).

Women perceived to be old are marginalized, bereft of power and may be subject to violence and exploitation (Laws, 1995). Gender and ageist stereotypes intertwine in old age, especially for women (Clarke & Griffin, 2008). In a double standard of aging (Sontag, 1972), the bodies of older women are reviled as unattractive, while older men's bodies are perceived as distinguished and as having character (Clarke & Griffin, 2008). With increasing promotion of individual responsibility for health, physical signs of aging are taken as evidence that a woman has not controlled her diet, actively exercised or lived an appropriate lifestyle. Sagging, wrinkling and greying are symbols of lack of control (Jones & Pugh, 2005), and they mark women, earlier than men, as "old" (Calasanti, 2007), leading to differential treatment for older women, who are judged as undeserving (Jones & Pugh, 2005). It is little wonder that aging women attempt to extend and prolong middle age by spending increasing amounts of time, money and effort to avoid the appearance of aging (Calasanti, 2007). Even though weight gain is normative in later life, older women frequently express discontent with their weight and the loss of their youthful appearance (Clarke & Griffin, 2008).

Staying fit and healthy in old age, the underpinnings of successful aging, is about not looking old and maintaining a youthful appearance (Calasanti, Slevin, & King, 2006). Women's bodies continue to be objectivized in old age (Clarke & Griffin, 2008). Images on television advertising old people playing golf or walking on the beach at sunset illustrate the successfully aged woman as slim, healthy, active, attractive and engaged in social relationships. In reality, older women's bodies as objects are judged as unattractive. In order to not be seen as old, women develop strategies to retain and maintain their youthfulness, such as undergoing cosmetic surgery and using lotions, creams and hair dyes to erase signs of aging (Calasanti, Slevin, & King, 2006). When women cannot maintain the healthy body expected of the successfully aging woman because of chronic conditions, they experience low self-esteem, a result of their deviation from youthful standards of beauty (Clarke & Griffin, 2008). Phrases used by women to deny their age, such as "I don't feel my age," are indicative of the power of youth to define old age (Gullette, 2004). The norms of youth and femininity continue to plague women as they age (Clarke & Griffin, 2008).

Productivity denotes social worth. Together with the perceived lack of productivity in unpaid domestic labour, this may serve to keep older women active longer in the paid workforce, where they are also devalued, yet economically productive. A lack of economic productivity renders women in later life dependent, since economic productivity is so closely linked to independence in our society. However, the focus on economic productivity renders invisible the contribution of older women to voluntary unpaid work, among other things. Independence stretches beyond the merely economic to the physical, social and emotional, about which many older women express a deep fear (Dillaway & Byrne, 2009). The successful aging discourse reinvigorates the fear of dependency with specificity — fear of aging with a disability (Angus & Reeve, 2006). In order to be productive, older women must first be, and remain, disease-free (Dillaway & Byrne, 2009).

Old age is perceived as unavoidably about disease and physical and mental decline, and therefore a natural part of growing older. As part of the natural order of things, it is used to justify limiting the rights and authority of women in later life (Calasanti, Slevin, & King, 2006; Sharpe, 1995). Loss of authority and autonomy result in, for example, older women's health complaints being taken less seriously by physicians (Robb, Chen, & Haley, 2002). Treating women in later life as children, for example, through the use of "baby talk," and discussing them with a caregiver or companion in their presence as though they were not there, minimizes and disrespects them (Sharpe, 1995). Their ability to make decisions about their health is undermined (Wilson, 2000). Dependency is created in a climate in which older women are seen as physically compromised and thought to be not competent to complete tasks themselves, often leading to a self-fulfilling prophecy. Perceived as contributing little to the social purse and as a drain on resources, older women are devalued as having little social worth (Kane, 2008). An aversion to older women by health professionals can result in humiliating health care encounters that compromise the quality of care (Sharpe, 1995).

Ageism is a tacit, unexamined assumption (Angus & Reeve, 2006), a subtle discrimination that may not be recognized by either health professionals or aging women (Sharpe, 1995). The implicit nature of ageism affects women in later life detrimentally, whether or not it is intended or recognized (Angus & Reeve, 2006), and quality of care may be diminished (Sharpe, 1995). As a consequence of ageism, women's complaints may be considered part of normal aging and thus not worthy of further attention (Adelman, Greene, Charon, et al. 1990), for example, disabilities may be rendered invisible by old age (Sanders, Donovan, & Dieppe, 2002). Stereotypes may lead to older women being seen, incorrectly, by health professionals as resistant to treatment that would benefit them (Kane, 2008). Assertive older women may be labelled "difficult" patients, thus affecting the care they receive. Anger is not permitted in women in later life (Woodward, 2002). The use of curative measures for life-threatening disease, such as breast cancer, decrease as women age. High technology options for heart disease, the leading cause of death in older women, are less likely to be pursued for older women compared to older men (Sharpe, 1995), and the attribution of women's complaints to psychological causes may contribute to misdiagnoses (Spitzer, 2005). Women are underrepresented as participants or subjects in health and pharmaceutical research (Sharpe, 1995). Studies have found that clinical encounters with women patients sixty-five and over are shorter (Radecki, Kane, Solomon, et al., 1988a) and that diagnostic tests are used less often as patients age (Radecki, Kane, Solomon, et al., 1988b). Many programs for older women are developed and provided by younger people based on the latter's ageist assumptions of what it is like to be old, as are policies directed toward aging well (Angus & Reeve, 2006).

Older women's resistance to old age stereotypes, especially those that promote a view of women as dependent, can have detrimental effects for women. Self-reliance represents independence and maturity, and its potential loss in the face of ageist stereotypes of dependency can result in women's stubborn denial of assistance in times of need (Clark, 1972; Angus & Reeve, 2006). On the other hand, the displacement of dependency with a normalizing view that elders be responsible for their own health (healthy and successful aging discourses) creates a different problem. Disability, frailty and even aging itself can be interpreted as a failure to age well and renders women's dependency, disability and death silent and invisible (Angus & Reeve, 2006).

Fragmented Performances

By framing the way we see things, discourses provide a normative horizon within which we recognize ourselves and others (Bassett & Graham, 2007). Norms of recognition govern what is humanly recognizable and who and what are recognized (Butler, 2001). The woman who conforms to the discourses of healthy and successful aging can, for a while, avoid being recognized as the dependent, disabled, difficult, lonely woman. She can hold old age temporarily at bay by maintaining a youthful appearance through transferring the work ethic to physical activity, undergoing cosmetic surgery and applying dyes and creams to her sagging, wrinkled and grey-haired body. Eventually, however, she will be seen by others and herself as described in the discourses: declining and dependent, physically and cognitively impaired. She will measure herself against the need to take responsibility and not be a burden on society and find herself wanting. The performance of old age by women is fragmented. Ageism and the discourses of successful and healthy aging are a pervasive form of oppression. Subtle, to the point of being little recognized, they operate at a tacit level to constitute the personhood of women in later life. Yet within this pervasive form of oppression, resistance is possible. The oppressive power of discourses is in their iteration and recitation (Butler, 1990). Only by being repeated over and over again do they have a normalizing effect. Yet the repetition is never perfect. Our accounts about ourselves are never consistent with one another. They break apart and are open to reinterpretation. It is in the partiality of the discourses we tell ourselves and others tell us that the possibility exists for making new discourses, new norms (Butler, 2001), devoid of ageism.

Race and Racism
as Determinants of Health

Josephine B. Etowa & Elizabeth A. McGibbon

The myth that Canada is a land in which human rights have always been protected and respected is so deeply engrained in the minds of Canadians that there is often a refusal to acknowledge that Canada has a racist history, which has been echoed in modern policies. However, Canada's racist past is readily observable, requiring only an overview of legislation that has been implemented in the course of Canada's history. (Roy, 2008, p. 1)

Racism harms the health and reduces the lifespan of millions of people who experience this oppression. Historical and current societal power imbalances mean that intersections of gender, race and social class have serious and enduring impacts on the health and well-being of people of colour in Canada (Calliste & Dei, 2000; Galabuzi, 2006; McGibbon & Etowa, 2009). For example, the poor health outcomes of Indigenous (First Nations, Inuit and Métis) peoples can best be traced to brutal treatment at the hands of White colonial imperialism, rather than deficits in lifestyle. Although lifestyle has an impact on health outcomes, only systemic anti-racist social change will improve the health outcomes of Indigenous peoples (McGibbon, 2008).

This chapter discusses race and racism as social determinants of health (SDH), including their intersections with other SDH such as gender, education and employment. We specify the logical links among these SDH to illuminate their complex interconnectedness and multiple impacts on health outcomes and health care access. We revisit the cycle of oppression, presented in Chapter 1, with a focus on the creation and maintenance of racism and the persistently poorer health outcomes of people of colour. An intersectionality lens, as described in Chapter 2, is emphasized, and we include further evidence of the synergies of various forms of oppression and their relationship to physical and mental health outcomes.

The evidence that race is a social determinant of health spans several decades and consistently points to race as central in the health and well-being of individuals, families, communities and nations. In order to address race and its impact on health and health care, it is imperative to discuss racism because this is what makes race salient. While genetic differences are important, such as the incidence of sickle cell anemia, health inequities of racialized peoples are rooted in systemic racism. For example, studies have compared hypertension rates of African-Americans with West Africans, who are genetically quite similar because most slaves were taken from this part of the world less than thirteen generations ago (Cooper & Rotimi 1997). These studies showed that West Africans have very little incidence of hypertension when compared with their American counterparts. While one might be tempted to attribute this difference to diet alone, there is ample evidence of the links between racism and cardiac outcomes (see Table 5.1).

Inequities based on the SDH, and identities related to gender and race have led to a growing recognition that health outcomes are linked to societal oppression and lack of entitlement to basic human and civil rights (McGibbon, 2009). Most vulnerable of all are people who experience intersecting disadvantages, including gender, racial discrimination and poverty. Women of colour routinely experience this triple jeopardy and its pernicious influence on their health (Bernard, 2002). Racial discrimination and other forms of intolerance infringe on the human rights and dignity of those who experience these injustices. It has thus become abundantly clear that inequities in health outcomes and health care cannot be reduced through medical and other health interventions alone.

Inscribing Racism on Body and Mind

There is little doubt that race, more accurately racism, determines health. The compromised mental and physical health outcomes of Indigenous peoples and peoples subject to translocation and slavery is well documented. First Nations people living on reserves have reported rates of heart disease that are 16 percent higher than the overall Canadian rate, and First Nations women and men have life expectancies that are 5.3 and 7.4 years shorter, respectively (Statistics Canada, 2001). Statistics also show that African American lung and cancer patients are less likely to receive chemotherapy (Earle, Venditti, Neuman, et. al. 2000) and unlikely to receive treatment for prostate cancer (Hoffman, Harlan & Klabunde, 2003). Black women are significantly less likely than White women to receive minimum expected therapy for breast cancer (Breen, Wesley, Merril, & Johnson, 2004). Evidence also suggests that Black women in Canada face similar barriers to appropriate care and experience health deficits that are similar to those of African American women. Although most available race-related population health and epidemiological research is from the United States, there is little reason to believe that these inequities are not present in Canada and elsewhere. Table 5.1 provides evidence of how oppression becomes inscribed on the body, mind and spirit

Table 5.1 Racism as a Social Determinant of Health: Health Outcomes and Access to Care*

Cancer: Breast & Cervical
- A Canadian study found that Aboriginal women who have experienced breast cancer must be made visible within health-care in a way that recognizes that their experiences are situated within the structural context of marginalization through colonial oppression (Poudrier & Mac-Lean, 2009).
- Among Black women aged less than 50 years, those who reported frequent everyday discrimination (e.g., being treated as dishonest) and major experiences of unfair treatment due to race (e.g., job, housing and police) were at statistically significantly higher risk for developing breast cancer than were women who reported infrequent experiences (Taylor, Williams, Makambi, et al., 2007).
- Ethnic minority women are diagnosed with more advanced disease and experience greater morbidity and mortality (Kim, Ashing-Giwa, Kagawa-Singer, et al., 2006).
- Black women are less likely than White women to be screened or to present with asymptomatic disease (Merkin, Stevenson, & Powe, 2002).

Cancer: Prostate
- African American men have higher morbidity, mortality and risk than Caucasians (Maliski, Connor, Fink, et al., 2006).
- African Americans with prostate cancer present with more advanced disease, and they have poorer survival rates than U.S. White men, even when diagnosed at the same stage (Oakley-Girvan, Kolonel, Gallagher, et al. 2003).

Cancer: Other
- First Nations adults in Canada have a 20.8% higher rate of cancer than the general Canadian population (Assembly of First Nations, 2007).
- African Americans are significantly less likely to receive major colorectal treatment for their cancer, follow-up treatment and chemotherapy (Cooper, Yuan, & Rimm, 2000).
- Members of visible minorities were less likely than White people to have been admitted to hospital, tested for prostate-specific antigen, administered a mammogram or given a pap test (Quan, Fong, De Coster, et al. 2006).

Cardio-Vascular
- Racism may increase risk for hypertension; these effects emerge more clearly for institutional racism than for individual level racism. All levels of racism may influence the prevalence of hypertension via stress exposure and reactivity and by fostering conditions that undermine health behaviours (Brondolo, Love, Pencille, et al., 2011).

Table 5.1 Racism as a Social Determinant of Health: Health Outcomes and Access to Care*
Cardio-Vascular (continued) • First Nations adults in Canada have a 7.6% rate of heart disease, compared to a 5.6% rate for the general population. High blood pressure is reported by 20.4% of First Nations adults, compared with 16.4% for the general population (Assembly of First Nations, 2007). • In patients undergoing coronary artery bypass surgery, being African American or Asian/Pacific Islander is significantly associated with being treated by surgeons of poorer quality, when quality is measured by risk-adjusted mortality rates (Rothenberg, Pearson, Zwanziger, et al. 2004). • In a U.S. study, researchers found that doctors' unconscious biases strongly influenced whether or not they gave the patients thrombolysis (a key treatment for coronary artery disease). As doctors' pro-White unconscious bias increased, so did their likelihood of treating White patients and not treating Black patients (Green, Carney, Pallin, et al. 2007). • As many as 30% of deaths of all Black men and 20% of deaths of all Black women are attributed to high blood pressure (American Heart Association, 2001). • Cardiovascular diseases are the leading cause of death in Black people (Enang, 2002).
Pain (Chronic and Acute) • African-Americans were more likely than Whites to report that they felt discriminated against in their ability to obtain care or treatment for their pain (Whites 9%, African-Americans 15%, Hispanics 13%). African-Americans males with low income were almost 3 times as likely as Whites to feel discriminated against in their efforts to obtain treatment for pain (27% vs 10%, respectively) (Nguyenlo, Ugarte, Fuller, et al. 2005). • In geographic settings with predominantly racial and ethnic minority patients, 62% of patients were undertreated by WHO standards, and they were three times more likely to be under-medicated than patients seen in non-minority settings (Green, Anderson, Baker, et al., 2003); • African American patients in nursing homes had a 63% greater probability of no pain treatment than non-Hispanic White patients. African American and Hispanic patients were less likely than non-Hispanic White patients to have pain reports documented in their charts (Green, Anderson, Baker, et al., 2003).
Diabetes • First Nations adults have almost four times the rate of diabetes than the general population (Assembly of First Nations, 2007). • Black women have more than twice the risk of developing adult-onset diabetes than White women. Black men have more than one and a half times the risk of developing diabetes (Brancati, Kao, Folsom, et al. 2000).

Table 5.1 Racism as a Social Determinant of Health: Health Outcomes and Access to Care*
Sickle Cell Anemia • Although sickle cell disease is not curable, early diagnosis would ensure appropriate management strategies, thereby reducing the number of deaths cause by the disease. Routine screening of Black newborns is an unrealized dream in Canada (Enang, 2002).
Please note: This table cites the terms used by the authors of the studies (i.e. Black, African American, Hispanic, Aboriginal, Ethnic Minority, Visible Minority, White, Caucasian, etc).

to create sustained health difficulties. Chapter 9 details the mental health threats of systemic racism.

How Do Race and Racism Determine Health?

Although race is universally applied as a stratification variable, race has absolutely no scientific meaning. Like national boundaries, the definitions of human races are strictly social constructions, evolving over time and space to accommodate the flow of human history. Our beliefs about race and its relationship to health and disease are influenced by the myth of innate racial differences that has evolved within our society (Kauffman & Cooper, 1996). Williams (1999: 176) defines race as "an ideology of inferiority that is used to justify unequal treatment (discrimination) of members of groups defined as inferior, by both individuals and societal institutions." Race has also been described as a social construction involving the classification of individuals into arbitrary groups and the assignment of disparate meaning and value to these constructed groups (Houston & Wood, 1996). Witzig (1996) confirms that race is a social construction created from prevailing social perceptions and without scientific evidence.

Racial classifications affect the personal, social, political and material circumstances of people's lives and consequently shape how they view themselves and others as well as their personal and societal relationships (Houston & Wood, 1996). Begley (1996: 68) states that the term race "can have a biological significance only when a race represents a uniform, closely inbred group, in which all family lines are alike — as in pure breeds of domesticated animals. These conditions are never realized in human types and impossible in large populations." *Mosby's Medical, Nursing and Allied Health Dictionary* defines race as "a vague unscientific term for a group of genetically related people who share some physical traits" (Glaze, Anderson and Anderson 1994: 657). According to Witzig, only 0.012 percent of the variation between humans in total genetic material can be attributed to differences in race.

Yet race is an emotionally laden word which evokes deep feelings and triggers stereotypical images about certain groups of people (Logan, Freeman & McRoy, 1990). Physical identity and social categorization, the essence of race, determine the predominant perceptions of people of colour in the Western world. For example, when people think of Black families, they immediately think of a racial group (Logan, Freeman, & McRoy, 1990). Although scientific evidence rejects the use of the social construct of race, it is still used in the health literature. Authors have even employed race "to attribute not only to physical characteristics, but also psychological and moral ones to members of given categories, thus justifying or naturalizing a discriminatory system" (Begley, 1996 p. 68). Systemic racism is common in society and arbitrary race groupings are part of this kind of racism (Witzig, 1996).

Shifting perspectives on the meaning of race notwithstanding, we cannot ignore the concept because we live in a society where race is one of the fundamental means of social categorization. Researchers cannot transcend these categories because there are no objective criteria for racial categorization other than "official" ones such as those used in the Canadian Census (e.g., visible minorities). It is equally important not to abandon these categories altogether because they capture important information about differences in disease risk and etiology. In addition, they help us to recognize the social reality of the associations between race and inequities in health and health care. The pathways through which racism affects health are shown in Figure 5.1, which illustrates how biased information, stereotyping, prejudice and discrimination interact within complex systemic webs to create and sustain oppressions such as racism, sexism, and classism.

Figure 5.1 Ruling Power Relations and the Cycle of Oppression

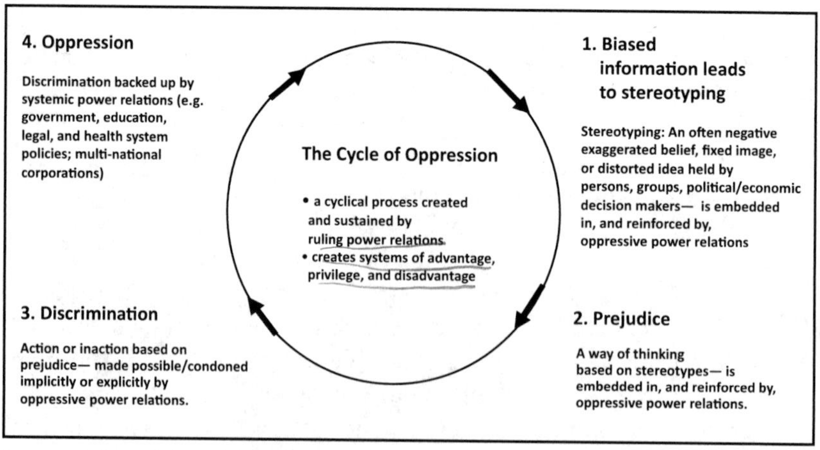

Source: *Adapted from McGibbon, Etowa & McPherson, 2008a.*

We all hold stereotypical views about individuals and groups of people. These stereotypes can lead to *thinking* in a particular way, which demonstrates prejudice. Henry, Tater and Mattis, et al. (2000) explicate common negative stereotypes of people of colour: Aboriginal people (savages, alcoholics, uncivilized, uncultured, murderers, noble, needing a White saviour, victim; Blacks (drug addicts, pimps, prostitutes, entertainers, athletes, drug dealers, murderers, gangsters, butlers and maids, simple-minded, savages, primitive, needing a White saviour); and Asians (untrustworthy, menacing, unscrupulous, submissive, maiming, quaint, gangsters, prostitutes, cooks, store vendors). These stereotypes lead to prejudicial thinking. When we then *act or fail to act* in a particular way, based on our prejudice, we participate in discrimination. For example, health care professionals are also immersed in these well known stereotypes. This stereotyping leads to inaction in the form of fewer specialist referrals for people of colour and disproportionately less follow-up treatment, as documented in this chapter.

When our discriminatory *actions or inactions are supported* or condoned by the health care system or other institutional structures, this process constitutes oppression. Although racism is demonstrated in individual and systemic actions or inactions, it is more deeply rooted at the systemic level because the power to make decisions, to take collective action and to allocate resources resides at this level (Enang, 2002). Systemic oppression is supported by policy action and inaction regarding persistently compromised health outcomes of people of color.

Racism at the systemic level manifests in material conditions and in access to power, including differential access to educational opportunities, health care and research resources (Etowa, Weins, Bernard, et al., 2007). Racism also includes interconnected factors of economic, environmental, psychosocial and iatrogenic (caused by hospitals and clinicians) conditions (Krieger, 2003). Table 5.2, which includes evidence from two qualitative studies in Canada, illustrates how systemic racism is articulated in everyday life.

Racism and Health: A Social Determinants Perspective

The concept of "determinants of health" provides a foundation for analysis of health and health care and the discovery of points for social action to address individual and systemic racism. Included in determinants of health are aspects of biologic and genetic endowment and social determinants. The social determinants of health, as laid out in the Toronto Charter (Raphael, 2009a) and as revised by Mikkonen and Raphael (2010), include early childhood development, employment and working conditions, income and its equitable distribution, food security, health care services, housing shortages, education, social exclusion, social safety nets, gender, age, race and Aboriginal status.

Table 5.2: Racism as a Social Determinant of Health: Voices from the Margins

Racism as Poison: "Racism in Canada is like slow poison… I see it as poison that invades the Black psyche, the Black experience… and unless we can get rid of that poison, we're not going to be totally healthy… It's insidious. It's slow. It's sly… It doesn't get you right away" (Etowa, 2005).

Racism as a Stress: "It [racism] causes certain amount of pressure and certain amount of stress… I used to suffer with severe migraine headaches." (Etowa, 2005).

Racism and Workplace Stress: "I was really close to suicide… I remember thinking to myself if I should take something, they'd probably revive me and I don't think I want to hang around here. It's just too stressful… I wasn't sleeping… I remember thinking… if I'm desperate to do this I'll just walk on the bridge and jump over it… That was what, we knew that's a real suicide, when you feel as if you really don't want to be revived. And because my head nurse was in psychiatry, I went to her and said, look, I am so desperate, I just feel like going down and jumping off the bridge… It was killing me. It was killing me" (Etowa, 2005).

The Impact of Racism: "They wanted to break me. They really wanted to break me. And they're very close to it, very, very close… I wasn't sleeping… And I found myself talking to myself when I was giving out pills… I was so stressed out…. I remember going on down the ward and… I would double check everything, because I was sort of spaced out. Somebody would tell me something, I'd have to go back over the phone number… it was stress 12 hours a day. I was sort of talking to myself to keep on doing things right" (Etowa, 2005).

Stereotypes and Quality of Care: "They were taking my blood. She got the student nurse to take my blood. But she couldn't find my vein. And she kept plucking around on me, and it was hurting me. So I told her, 'No, you can't keep doing this.' And the nurse said, 'No just try it one more time.' I said 'No, you're not trying it no more. Why can't you do it?' She said, 'Well, it's known that Black people have tougher skin than White people'" (Enang, 1999).

Curriculum Content and Lack of Diversity: "We need more of our people in the health care professions. And if it means we're going to have to start fighting to allow our young people into medical school, then we'll have to start doing that. I think that we need to attack some of the training institutions for change in their curriculum and in their approach. Then we need to attack our school, especially high schools and elementary schools, to get some mentors into the schools to encourage children to go into health care professions" (Enang, 1999).

Source: Enang [Etowa] (1999); Etowa (2005).

Historically, it has largely been assumed that differences in the health of people of colour were due to differences in biologic and genetic endowment — the biophysical attributes which are inherited from our parents or acquired throughout our lifespan. It is now well recognized that biologic and genetic endowment, although very important in determining health, are not the major determinants of the health of individuals, families, communities and nations (Raphael, 2004). Rather, health inequities have been closely linked with differences in social, economic, cultural and political circumstances. Economic inequities, in particular, have been implicated in poor health: people with fewer economic resources are at much greater risk of illness and are much less likely to have timely access to health and social services (Galabuzi, 2006). Differences in income levels and socioeconomic status (SES) demonstrate the continued primacy of material influences on health (Wilkinson & Marmot, 2005). Inadequate household income for securing healthy food creates nutritional deficits, which greatly impact health and development across the lifespan. When families lack access to basic essentials, such as food, education and safe shelter, their health is compromised.

Health inequities along racial lines have been created and reinforced by limited access to educational and employment opportunities for minority groups through processes such as segregation (McGibbon & Etowa, 2009). Racial differences in SES have been well documented in the literature, and health researchers examining the association between race and health routinely adjust for this variable (Krieger, 2003; Williams, 1999). Thus, SES is not only considered a cofounder of racial differences in health but "part of the causal pathways by which race affects health" (Williams, 1999, p. 177). Race is therefore an antecedent and a determinant of SES, and racial differences in SES are to some degree a reflection of the implementation of discriminatory policies and practices premised on the inferiority of certain racial groups (Williams, 1999). Krieger (1987) argues that the poorer health of Black people relative to the White population is the result of White privilege, enforced through slavery and other forms of racial discrimination, rather than innate inferiority. Furthermore, Krieger (2003: 195) states that "health is harmed not only by heinous crimes against humanity, such as slavery, lynching and genocide, but also by the grinding economic and social realities of what Essed (1991) has aptly termed, 'everyday racism.'"

As detailed in Chapter 2, the SDH intersect with identities such as race, social class and gender to produce a powerful synergy of disadvantage for racialized peoples. For example, gender intersects with race to cause a higher rate of unemployment among immigrant, Indigenous and African Canadian women (Galabuzi, 2006; Statistics Canada, 2006b, 2006c). Poverty has been directly linked to decreased access to health care and decreased health outcomes. Here the intersections of age, race, gender and SDH such as employment and income combine to limit health care access. Immigrant women of colour, who earn less than the Canadian average for women, face additional barriers related to geography, since their extended families are often far away and many immigrant individuals and families lack the resources to maintain connections with their country of origin. Senior Canadians are at particular risk, regardless of gender, race or ethnicity, since home care, or family care, is becoming medical support "on the cheap." Family members, usually women, have taken on the additional burden of home care. Pan American Health Organization director Mirta Periago (2004) asked the following question at an international gathering in Washington: "What would happen if all the women of the world decided to go on strike and for just one day refused to provide health care in their homes and communities? What would be the catastrophic implications for global well-being?"

Most women of colour experience all the major forms of oppression, including classism, racism and sexism. A close examination of the United States 1990 census revealed that 34 percent of Black women were living below poverty line compared to 11 percent of White women (Krieger, Rowley, Herman et al., 1993). More than fifteen years later, these figures were mirrored in a Canadian study of Black women in rural communities. Among the participants who responded to the income question, a significant 72 percent earned less than $15,000 in average annual personal income and 45 percent earned less than $15,000 in average annual household income, which is well below the national and provincial poverty lines. These statistics revealed that a considerable proportion of Black families in these communities were very low-income earners. Income remains an important measure and an integral determinant of the SES of individuals, families and communities, and there is a strong relationship among income, other health determinants and health status (Etowa, Weins, Bernard, et al., 2007)

Galabuzi (2006) has written extensively about the interconnections among racism, social exclusion, unemployment, underemployment, individual and family income, and education. As Canada enters a new century, racialized people continue to experience stark inequities related to each of these SDH. The income gap between racialized and non-racialized earners continues to be an important indicator of racial inequality in Canada, as demonstrated by unemployment, labour-market participation and employment income (2006). Galabuzi reports that employment income for racialized people was 15 percent lower than the national average, for racialized women, the inequity is even greater — their average earnings in 1996 were $16,621, compared to $23,635 for racialized men, $19,495 for other women and $31,951 for other men. In terms of education, the proportion of racialized group members achieving post-secondary degrees is growing at a higher rate than in the general population. Yet there has not been a corresponding increase in employment or income. So what factors cause this discrepancy? As Galabuzi (2006: 111) points out, the discrepancy suggests an 'x,' or unknown, factor: "We suggest that this 'x' factor is the devaluation of the human capital of racialized group members, resulting from racial discrimination in the labor market."

Inequities in the sdh combine to amplify systemic threats to the health of people of colour. The gap in the low-income rate between recent immigrants and Canadian-born individuals has widened significantly in recent decades. In 1980, low-income rates among immigrants who had arrived between 1975 and 1980 were 1.4 times those of people born in Canada. In 1990, low-income rates among immigrants who arrived between 1985 and 1990 were 2.1 times those of the Canadian-born, and by 2000, low-income rates among recent immigrants were 2.5 times those of the Canadian-born (Statistics Canada, 2003). Statistics Canada defines recent immigrants as those who arrived in Canada during the five years before the census in question. Immigrants of colour have the compounding burden of racism, which makes their incomes even less, on average, than the general population of immigrants in Canada.

Racism and Barriers in Access to Care

An increase in acute care health services does not necessarily improve population health. However, in the debate about the salience of health care as an sdh, there is often a failure to analyze barriers in access. When individuals and families access health care they arrive with more than their immediate physical and mental health concerns. The intersections of their identities (e.g., age, gender, race, social class) and intersections of their social determinants of health (e.g., early childhood development, employment) are inextricably linked to their health concerns. Statistics in the previous section provide foundational evidence for the direct and often devastating relationship between these intersectionalities and inequities in access to health care. For example, the vast majority of health care in Canada is provided with the assumption that individuals and families can afford costs currently considered peripheral: transportation, prescription medications, over-the-counter antibiotics and anti-inflammatory drugs, orthopedic braces, time away from work, child care and so on. Adequate employment and income has thus become a prerequisite for full health care access and optimal health, particularly for rural, remote and northern Canadians (McGibbon, 2009).

Health care access then becomes a powerful determinant of health by virtue of its policy-based neutrality, or the presumptuousness regarding the hidden costs of full access, and its employment-neutral stance regarding which Canadians can, or cannot, afford access and health maintenance costs. When individuals and families cannot afford to follow up on recommended

Table 5.3: Barriers in Access to Health Services for Rural Aboriginal and African Canadians	
Barriers: Health Service Providers	Barriers: The Agency, The System
Racial profiling in the health system: Aboriginal, Black people treated differently, less competently — related to systemic racism, racist attitudes of providers, White privilege. **Cultural literacy, health literacy:** lack of culturally appropriate health information, tendency for health workers to not care to give available information. **Resulting lack of safe services:** people not offered available care, not assessed in a timely manner when compared to White counterparts, lack of personal attention from providers, a habit of ignoring the concerns of Aboriginal and Black people, thus incompetent care. **Lack of communication at entry point:** insulting questions based on stereotypes: "When was your last drink?"; barriers related to stereotypical attitudes; language of service providers not the same as that of consumers.	**Services are "streamlined":** economically efficient but ineffective because they are too fragmented, i.e., when there are three doctors, yet no continuity of care (service providers not communicating with each other). **People and families are pushed into partnerships** based on government department organization rather than needs; lack of support from politicians in the advocacy process. **Power without accountability:** provincial professional organizations must be held accountable for racist actions — forced to uphold a code of ethical conduct; need more openly transparent professional organizations and governments. The current system does not provide a reliable method; 'How can you hire a fox to look after the chickens?' In provincially funded health, social services, when something goes wrong in a person's care, there is often a one-sided investigation of complaints, often with no offer of explanation, accountability or compassion.

Table 5.3: Barriers in Access to Health Services for Rural Aboriginal and African Canadians	
Insensitivity: need cultural sensitivity/cultural competence education in health system and education of health providers: not just the learning of skills — need to change values; training especially needed in rural areas where providers become comfortable having the privilege of "saying what they want." Training must be anti-racist, human rights oriented.	**Barriers in the legal system:** when people try to hold services responsible, lawyers may be in a conflict of interest due to personal relationships in the health, social services system, especially in rural areas.

Long term care options not available to First Nations persons on reserves, especially in the area of mental health. |
| **Communities used for experimentation** in terms of treatments, including over-prescription. This must be addressed, changed. | **Families are left to struggle on their own,** without resources when trying to navigate the system; need advocates from the community. |
| **Service provision is not reflective of the community,** in ways of health care provision and in lack of Aboriginal and Black providers.

The effects of the intersection of race, class and gender need to be considered re: how service providers treat people, respond to their needs "to be a woman, a Black woman, and an ordinary Black woman." Service providers are unable or unwilling to provide proper, compassionate care unless you demonstrate some sort of privilege, i.e., being a professor. | **Questioning people in power, authority is very difficult,** takes much energy, resilience, support, yet it is so important because you or your family members will die if you don't speak up. Obtaining safe care is very difficult, energy draining; need to become more skilled at fighting a system that is prone to retaliation.

There is tremendous stress associated with advocacy struggles and the process of overcoming these barriers; individuals and families are sometimes punished for bringing advocacy issues to light. |

Source: *McGibbon, Calliste, Arbuthnot, Bassett, Cameron, Graham and MacDonald 2008.*

treatments due to lack of money, they are at risk of being labelled "non-compliant" and thus having their health problems blamed on their lack of initiative. As evidenced in this chapter, lack of affordability is related to age, gender, race and social class. Canada now has 15.5 percent of children living in relative poverty, defined as households with incomes below 50 percent of the national median, thus ranking seventeenth out of twenty-three developed countries (UNICEF, 2005). Table 5.3 reports important barriers in access to health services for Aboriginal and African Canadians, underscoring the embeddedness of racism and the urgent need for systemic change.

These barriers in access are woven into the health care system, which is itself grounded in medical imperialism. For example, Black people are subjected to insensitive or inappropriate care when their illnesses are interpreted as the consequence of inherent predispositions to violence or sexual promiscuity (Bernard, 2002; Utsey, Ponterotto, Reynolds, et al., 2000) or from subtler assumptions embedded in the health care system, particularly the tendency to embrace White, middle-class, male experience as normative. The health indicators assessed in the Apgar test, used to assess health of newborn babies, for example, is derived from assessment of White newborns. This process makes the Apgar assessment of the skin color of the Black newborn much less useful (Enang, 2002).

In the health fields, cultural competence is the main approach to addressing these individual and systemic barriers in access for racialized persons and groups. Although initiatives related to cultural competence have fostered cross-cultural health care and created a mutual ground to initiate a dialogue about issues of difference, a critical analysis of racial issues and an understanding of the macro-level workings of the health care system are necessary to design and implement much needed policy changes to ensure truly accessible health services for racialized and marginalized peoples. Although health literature suggests that there is a need for health care professionals to understand and adapt to cultural diversity through culturally competent care, proponents of anti-racism have argued that professionals must challenge racism, rather than opting for the politically soft option that merely reifies culture (Alleyne, Papadopoulos, & Tilki, 1994). These authors further note that such an approach denies the centrality or existence of racism and pays "superficial attention to cultural rites and rituals" (583).

Models of cultural competence fall short on a number of counts. Following years of efforts to implement such models in health care, there remains minimal evidence to demonstrate its effectiveness in improving health outcomes or reducing health inequities (McGibbon & Etowa, 2009). Drevdahl, Canales and Dorcy (2008: 20) illustrate the problem with cultural competence with an analogy: "Cultural competence is like a goldfish tank in the centre of the hospital waiting room. It improves the atmosphere and helps patients relax; however, it does not eliminate the actual problem that brought the patients into the hospital in the first place."

In contrast, the term "cultural safety" is now in common usage among anti-racist health and social services practitioners. The concept of cultural safety (*kawa whakaruruhau*) appeared in a formal sense in New Zealand in the early 1990s, when it was used to describe a more focused cultural response to power imbalances between health professionals and the recipients of health care, and Maori recipients in particular (Woods, 2010). Cultural safety has subsequently been perceived as a guide for responding to the health problems of many of the world's most vulnerable or marginalized ethnic groups (Woods). Cultural safety is distinguished from cultural competence in its explicit attention to oppression, imperialism, post-colonialism and White privilege (McGibbon, Didham, Smith, et al., 2009)

A cultural safety approach holds great promise for disrupting racism in the health fields and elsewhere, even with the complex challenge of integrating this way of being and thinking into practice, research, education and policy-making. Racism has been increasingly implicated in known disparities in the health and health care of racial, ethnic and cultural minorities groups. Despite the obvious ethical implications of this observation, racism as an ethical issue *per se* has been relatively neglected in health care ethics discourse (Johnstone & Kanitsaki, 2010). In a society that is increasingly multicultural, there is now a movement, albeit small, among health practitioners, educators, researchers and policymakers to reframe racism as a moral issue in health care:

> Such changes demand a greater awareness and responsiveness to-wards the cultural differences between each individual and/or groups of individuals, and especially the shared beliefs and practices of various minority social, ethnic, religious and gender groups in society, such as young people, elderly people, and those who are mentally ill or disabled. However, the values, ideals and basic rights of such groups have often been overlooked, ignored or minimized because, as is common in western or postcolonial countries, any arguments from a cultural or ethically relativist perspective are often overridden to favour those of the more prevalent views of western ethnocentrism and moral universality. (Woods, 2010, p. 718)

Conclusions

The evidence of racism as a social determinant of heath requires not only an understanding of biologic and genetic endowment, but a consistent focus on the threat of racism. Racism as a process and an outcome overlays all other health determinants for people of colour. The way forward lies in sustained attention to the foundations of racism, including White privilege, Eurocentric biomedical hegemony and modern-day post-colonial repetitions of historical imperialism. In Canada we have barely begun a truth and reconciliation process about Canada's legacy of slavery and genocide. This chapter focuses on some of these antecedents of the markedly different health outcomes of people of colour, compared to White people. We provide core ideas for understanding the how and the why of these health inequities. Although there has been little attention to post-colonial theory in the health fields (Anderson, 2000), a sustained focus on oppression and structural power is surely the path to reducing the human and financial costs of continued racism.

• 6 •

Oppression and the Health
of Indigenous Peoples

Marie Battiste &
James [Sa'ke'j] Youngblood Henderson

The endless cycles of foreign diseases and colonial and racial oppression have generated a fragile mind, spirit and body of Indigenous peoples (Battiste, 2000; Dressler, 2000; Henderson, 2007; Kunitz, 1994; Royal Commission on Aboriginal People, 1996). Indigenous peoples are a political and social construct, not a racial or ethnic reality. They have extraordinary variation in their lifestyles, traditions and cultures, and as such, there is no single clear definition of Indigenous peoples. They exist within ancient relationships within defined territories and are distinctive in knowledge and language and law of life (Henderson, 2007). They are many diverse peoples who occupy certain environments and retain diverse traditions and laws, although most, if not all, have suffered intergenerational trauma because of their heritage and lifeways under colonialism, oppression, Eurocentric development and forced assimilation under state educational policies. After centuries of oppression, there are some 5000 Indigenous peoples around the world — with a total population of about 300 million, representing around 4 percent of the global population (Howitt, 1996).

Notwithstanding changes in statistical definitions and variable practices of enumeration among and between Indigenous peoples that make comparisons difficult, inequalities in health status are an important measure of the quality of the health system. Within developed countries, in almost all cases, Indigenous peoples generally have lower health indices and lower life expectancy than non-Indigenous peoples in the same territory and a higher incidence of most diseases (e.g., diabetes, mental disorders, cancers), including a higher experience of what are now considered Third World diseases (e.g., tuberculosis, rheumatic fever) (Kunitz 1994). Chapter 5 details more of these oppression-related inequities in health outcomes.

Although the standards of health of Indigenous peoples show differences, spiritually connected similarities exist in their worldviews and their relationships to their land and to each other, as well as in their exposure to colonization, racism, discrimination and oppression. These similarities are revealed in their patterns of disease, health determinants and health care strategies. For example, beginning in the fifteenth century, the First Nations of North and South America, and continuing in the eighteenth and nineteenth centuries, groups as diverse as Maori in New Zealand, Australian Aborigines, native Hawaiians and the Saami and Inuit of the Arctic suffered greatly and were nearly decimated by importation of infectious diseases by Europeans, including measles, typhoid fever, tuberculosis and influenza (Durie, 1998). By the mid-twentieth century, however, following the near universal experience of being displaced and becoming urban refugees, other health risks emerged. While communicable diseases continue to affect large Indigenous populations, vulnerability to injury, alcohol and drug misuse, cancer, heart disease, kidney disease, obesity, suicide and diabetes have become the modern Indigenous health hazards (Cunningham & Condon, 1996; Seear, 2007).

Leaving aside the damaging views of early colonists about "primitive," "backward" and "deficit" peoples (Havemann, 1999), explanations for current Indigenous health status, usually derived from Eurocentric methods (Amin, 1988; Blaut, 1993), can be grouped into the following themes: oppression and related stress; racialization and disparities of health care, training and education of Indigenous populations; genetic vulnerability; and forced cognitive assimilation. From an Indigenous perspective, these themes are overlapping and can be conceptualized as a causal continuum of oppression. At one end are "short distance" factors, such as the continued use of a false concept of race and genetics in the scientific and health communities, which masks the impacts of oppression on the bodies of Indigenous peoples. At the other end are "long distance" factors, including health consequences arising from government policies. Values, lifestyles, standards of living and culture, so important to clinical understandings, lie midway.

These themes have led to fragile consciousnesses, poor health, socio-economic disadvantage and resource alienation among Indigenous peoples. Poor housing, low educational achievement, unemployment and inadequate incomes are known to correlate with a range of ways of living that predispose populations to disease and injury (National Health Committee, 1998). These socioeconomic disadvantages are central to the contemporary health and experience of Indigenous peoples. Alienation from natural resources, along with environmental degradation, have also been identified as a cause of poor health. Similarly, cultural alienation has been recognized as an important consideration in creating effective health care (Duran & Duran, 1995). Health workers are more familiar with short and mid-distance factors, but improving the health of Indigenous peoples requires a holistic approach covering a wide spectrum of interventions, including "long distance" factors related to public policy. When doctor and health professional and patient are from different cultural backgrounds, the issue of cultural safety arises, and the likelihood of misdiagnosis and non-compliance is greater.

The World Health Organization Geneva Declaration (WHO, 1999) on the Health and Survival of Indigenous Peoples proposed the following definition of Indigenous health:

> Indigenous peoples' concept of health and survival is both a collective and an individual inter-generational continuum encompassing a holistic perspective incorporating four distinct shared dimensions of life. These dimensions are the spiritual, the intellectual, the physical, and the emotional. Linking these four fundamental dimensions, health and survival manifests itself on multiple levels where the past, present, and future co-exist simultaneously.

The Geneva Declaration recommends several strategies, including capacity building, research, cultural education for health professionals, increased funding and resources for Indigenous health, a reduction in the inequities accompanying globalization and constitutional and legislative changes by states. In their Declaration of the Rights of Indigenous Peoples (United Nations, 2007a), the World Health Assembly and the United Nations General Assembly resolved to urge member states to recognize and protect the right of Indigenous people to the highest attainable standard of health and to make adequate provisions for Indigenous health needs, while respecting and maintaining traditional healing practices and remedies.

Many Indigenous peoples have emphasized autonomy, self-determination and human rights. They have given priority to developing an Indigenous health workforce that has both professional and cultural competence. They have also promoted the adoption of Indigenous health perspectives, including spirituality, in conventional Eurocentric health services. Traditional healing practices have been suggested as a further strategy, though generally as part of comprehensive primary health care and in collaboration with health professionals (Warry, 1998; Hill, 2003). However, while access to quality integrated health care, including traditional healing practices, is important, removing oppression and trauma may have greater potential for improving and sustaining the highest possible health for Indigenous peoples.

The Impact of Psychosocial Stress

Although oppression has been discussed since at least the eighteenth century, oppression-related stress is a relatively new concept. Psychosocial stress has now become one of the most ubiquitous concepts in scientific health and contemporary discourses. Since the 1960s, a plethora of disciplines including psychology, psychiatry, nursing, medicine, sociology, anthropology and pharmacology have studied psychosocial stress (Mulhall, 1996). In the twenty-first century alone, more than 100,000 articles have been indexed in PubMed with the keyword *stress*. This veritable mountain of research has been accompanied by a profusion of conceptual approaches, which as a whole, suffer from difficulties in characterizing stress (Hinkle, 1987; Quick, Nelson, Quick, et al., 2001).

Despite this profusion of research and thought, sparse information exists on the relationships among oppression, stress and health for Indigenous peoples. What has not been made overtly clear, in the face of the dire statistics on Indigenous peoples and health, is that colonial policy, bureaucracies and institutions have created the crisis in their health, rather than the biology and culture of Indigenous peoples themselves. Colonial health policies have always resided in the false assumptions of race science: that Indigenous peoples were biologically predetermined to vanish, that they were inherently inferior and deficient, and that their culture caused them to pursue deleterious lifestyles and to be unhealthy (Lux, 2001). In addition, past and present education systems that have attempted to forcibly assimilate Indigenous peoples to colonial modes have generated multi-generational oppression and trauma. These processes of cognitive assimilation have generated many soul wounds (Duran & Duran, 1995) and diseases within Indigenous peoples. It is well accepted that the forced education of Indigenous peoples was a substantial contributor to the current high levels of suicide, substance abuse and family violence among residential school survivors.

Racialization

From the earliest thoughts about colonialism, the racialization of Indigenous people has preoccupied Eurocentrism (Chesterman & Galligan, 1998; Gardiner-Garden, 2003; McCorquodale, 1997). Historical approaches to defining Indigeneity focused on the need to survey and control socialization, mobility and biological reproduction (Dodson, 1994), while contemporary constructions of Indigeneity are primarily concerned with attributing the cause of Indigenous inequality to the deviant and "othered' Indigene (Brough, 1999; Cunneen, 2001). Furthermore, public health research is deeply implicated in such racialization of Indigenous peoples, both historically (Anderson, 2002) and in present-day research (Bond, 2005; Humphery, 2001; Smith, 1999). As a consequence of racializing practices, Indigenous peoples are subject to racism in the political domain (Augoustinos, Tuffin, & Rapley, 1999); health (Henry, Tater, Mattis, et al., 2000) and education systems (Battiste, 2000); sport (Gorman, 2004); the legal and criminal justice systems (Cunneen, 2001; Royal Commission on Aboriginal Peoples 1995); and civil society as a whole (Cowlishaw, 1997; Goodstone, Quayle, & Ranald, 2001; Hollinsworth, 1998; Human Rights and Equal Opportunity

Commission 1991; Lattas, 2001; Mellor, 2003). The breadth and depth of these systemic racializing practices has had an enduring negative impact on Indigenous peoples.

Racism should be conceptualized as one of the many types of oppression that Indigenous peoples have had to endure. It is an ideology about essentializing people to groups (Paradies, 2007; Miles & Brown, 2003) based on phenotype, ancestry and/or culture and creating differences between groups that are embodied in attitudes, beliefs, behaviours, laws, norms and practices (Memmi, 1969). This cognitive process is called racialization and covers unconscious, systemic forms and intentional acts. Such population descriptors have been shown time and again to be historically and situationally determined, unreliable and imprecise proxies for human genetic differences. Nevertheless, racialization continues to occur when population descriptors are used as *de facto* markers of biological differences between human groups. When inequalities of morbidity and mortality are explained or hypothesized as a condition of innate and fixed genetic differences, the existence of sociopolitical inequalities and oppression among human groups are effectively denied, and embodied health outcomes are attributed to these putative biological differences.

Racial identity is best understood as a marker of social relationship rather than as an unalterable individual trait (Lopez, 1994; Zuberi, 2001). In contemporary society, as in the past, the attribution of race to individuals often depends on the presence of particular morphological characteristics, such as skin colour, as well as known or assumed lines of descent from ancestors with particular morphological characteristics or defined geographic ancestry (Berg, Bonham, Boyer, et al., 2005). The continuously varying character of such features in human populations, combined with the historically and culturally contingent nature of attaching social meaning to specific morphologies, explains the marked variation in the number, nature and type of races identified over both time and space (Brodkin, 2000).

In contemporary health care, race science and racism categories are perpetuated through the concept of geneticization, the notion that genes are the primary determinants of biology and behaviour (Lippman, 1993), despite the fact that humans are remarkably genetically similar, sharing 99.9 percent of their genomes in common (Li & Sadler, 1991; Stephens, Schneider, Tanguay, et al., 2001). Existing racial categories are common, rather than biologically distinct. However, Eurocentric categories of race or ethnicity are constructed on the small intra-species diversity of 0.1 percent among humans. Approximately 10–15 percent of the genetic variations are found between these Eurocentric categories of groups; and 85–90 percent of genetic variations occur within socially constructed "groups" (Romualdi, Balding, Nasidze, et al., 2002).

Despite what is best recognized as a largely arbitrary system of Eurocentric classification of peoples laid atop complex geographic patterns of population genetic variation, recent research has assigned individuals to likely racial (or, as they are often designated, ancestral) backgrounds by a cumulative examination of differences in the frequencies of common genetic variants, as well as more geographically restricted (i.e., population-specific) polymorphisms (Rothenberg, Pearson, Zwanziger, et al., 2002). Genetic causes have been investigated in diabetes, alcohol-related disorders and some cancers for Indigenous peoples, although they are generally regarded as less significant than oppression and socioeconomic factors.

Although most health-related genetic research has been conducted on populations of European ancestry (Ioannidis, Ntzani, Trikalinos, et al., 2004), the presentation of genetic findings using folk taxonomies of ethnicity or race reinforces the fallacy that they are meaningful genetic categories. Indigenous people, in Third and Fourth World contexts, are often considered to be genetically susceptible to a plethora of chronic diseases (Cooper, Kaufman, & Ward 2003). Genetic explanations for ill-health are proposed when no such data are available, on the basis of nonsignificant findings or even when genetic variation is unrelated to the disease under study. The association between unsubstantiated genetic attributions and the social status of a racial group (Cooper, Kaufman, & Ward 2003) demonstrates the potential harm that may result from the continuing and increasing use of racial categories in genetic research (Ellison & Jones, 2002). To correct these erroneous and destructive assumptions, which emerge as oppression, Indigenous health issues have to be addressed from the vantage point of Indigenous knowledge, which affirms the holistic perspective of health as a basic human right. In Canada, this approach to health is not advocacy or an optional discussion — it is the innovative part of the constitutional order of Canada (Boyer, 2003). This rights-based analysis is further taken up in Chapter 13.

Researchers must conceptualize the effects of oppression and stress on Indigenous peoples in a clear and unambiguous manner in the models proposed, whether Eurocentric or Indigenous. The various types of stressors considered, and the contextual factors relevant to the stress process, must be clarified. This clarification is a necessary prerequisite to elucidating the complex relationships among health sequelae and outcomes, racism, oppression, stressors and Indigenous peoples under assimilation, colonialization and postcolonialism. Additionally, the studies or models must highlight the need to better understand the role of stressors in pathopsychological processes and in modifying health behaviours; the relationship between types of stressors and emotion/meaning focused coping strategies; the possibility that stressors may have differential effects on various physiological systems and may vary in their importance by social location (e.g., ethnicity, race and gender), both psychologically and behaviourally as well in the physiological pathways through which they operate; and the interplay between genotypical and phenotypical influences on both stress sequelae and exposure/responses to stressors.

Neocolonization and Eurocentric Analytical Systems

Several writers have drawn a link between oppression, colonization and the related stress and health disparities of Indigenous peoples (Cohen, 1999). They argue that loss of Indigenous sovereignty, along with dispossession of lands, waterways and customary laws, has created a climate of material and spiritual oppression with increased susceptibility to disease and injury. Bonnie and Eduardo Duran (Duran & Duran, 1995) have emphasized the relationship between oppression and soul wounds in Indigenous peoples. Their experience with Eurocentric analytical systems in health and medicine led them to conclude that the system is in desperate need of new descriptions and explanations for many of the illnesses that plague Indigenous peoples and that the Eurocentric system of disease conceptualization and treatment is inadequate for many of these problems. Although there are many programs and approaches to deal with the health and healing of Indigenous people, clinically speaking, these programs are inadequate. This is because once the pathology is neutralized in one aspect of the system, another area of the system will begin to show symptoms.

Duran and Duran (1995) also noted that the use of analytic systems of Eurocentric health and psychology have failed to heal these wounded peoples. The authors argue that these systems have continued the epistemic violence from which Native American communities have been suffering for many generations. They believe, in the future, that it will be beneficial to Indigenous peoples if the *Diagnostic Statistical Manual for Mental Disorders* (American Psychiatric Association, 2004) takes into account some of the issues of their historical and daily oppression. Diagnostic criteria such as acute or chronic reaction to genocide, colonialism, assimilation, racism and stress should exist. Without these categories there will be little honesty in Eurocentric health and healing practices with Indigenous peoples, and the ongoing epistemic violence will continue under the guise of contemporary health and healing systems, which will in fact be an ongoing attempt to control the lifeworld of Indigenous peoples (Duran & Duran, 1995). Eurocentric health professions must acknowledge that there are legitimate forms of generating Indigenous knowledge in the Indigenous communities and that this knowledge is valid in its own right, standing alongside that of other cosmologies (Duran & Duran). Unless Eurocentric health systems are reformulated in a manner in which Indigenous science, humanities and treatment strategies can flourish in an integrated trans-systemic synthesis, there will continue to be lack of efficacy from these Western systems of healing.

Paradies (2006b) has shown clear evidence that psychosocial stress is a risk factor for the development of a range of chronic diseases (Brunner, 1997; Brunner & Marmot, 2006; Cassidy, 1999; Brave Heart, 1999). It is also well known that Indigenous peoples are exposed to higher levels of stress and suffer a particularly high burden of chronic disease morbidity and mortality when compared to dominant members of their respective societies (Australian Bureau of Statistics & Australian Institute of Health and Welfare, 2005; Bramley, Hebert, Tuzzio, et al., 2005; Dressler, 2000; Kunitz, 1994).

Conclusion

Oppression and stress generate a complex determinant of health of Indigenous peoples. While a plethora of research on pyschosocial stress and health has been undertaken, it is surprising that there is very little empirical research about the association between stress and chronic disease for Indigenous peoples. Few evaluations of interventions to reduce stress, or its ill effects for Indigenous peoples, are documented in the published literature. Because a review of this very small body of existing research would be of dubious utility, little evidence exists for linking psychosocial stress to the development of chronic disease or the complication of its management for Indigenous peoples. Chapter 2 describes the relationship between oppression-related stress and health outcomes in an effort to more explicitly discuss this complex process.

The ways in which these factors can affect the relationship between stress and health for members of oppressed racial groups are complex. Clearly, further research on stress moderators is needed, as is the measurement and analysis of those moderating factors that have already been identified. The differential strength of association between stress and mental versus physical health corresponds to the findings for racism and raises similar questions about the mechanisms by which stress affects health. This relationship suggests the need for further research on the possible pathopsychological and/or neurophysiological aspects of the stress process that lead to ill health for oppressed racial groups, including Indigenous peoples. It is important to recognize racism as a significant determinant of health for Indigenous peoples and at the same time review institutional and legal anti-racism policies which could be implemented in an attempt to both reduce racism and oppression against Indigenous peoples and ameliorate its ill effects.

Social Exclusion as a Determinant of Health

Grace-Edward Galabuzi

In this chapter, I discuss the role social exclusion plays as a determinant of health outcomes and in generating health disparities among groups in society. The World Health Organization (WHO, 2003) has identified social exclusion as one of ten key social determinants of health (SDH), and according to Raphael (2009a), social exclusion is one of twelve such determinants of health. Social exclusion is manifest through forms of oppression that order institutional arrangements and power relations with the effect of marginalizing particular groups in society. It occurs through structural and historical processes that systematically generate social inequalities, resulting in enduring health disparities. International and Canadian research shows that groups experiencing various forms of oppression and social marginalization tend to sustain higher health risks and lower health status (WHO, 2003; Raphael, 2004; The Standing Senate Committee on Social Affairs, Science and Technology, 2009). Processes of feminization, racialization, colonization and displacement, among others, represent forms of oppression that have historically created unequal access to society's resources and to the health care system, giving rise to unequal health outcomes. This chapter explores the prevalence and impact of these processes on the health of groups and individuals.

First I introduce the concept of social exclusion and its implications for health outcomes, particularly for the social groups most affected. I discuss some examples of the various dimensions of exclusion — economic exclusion, spatial exclusion and the intersection of exclusion, poverty and health. Using examples of affected groups, such as women, racialized groups, Aboriginal peoples and immigrants, I address the impacts of differential economic, social and political relations arising from oppressions and leading to differential life chances and health outcomes. I suggest that these differential outcomes arise from the way these oppressions impose differential access to society's resources and relations of power. We see these oppressions as part of a complex set of structural imperatives that determine how society is organized through key institutional arrangements that shape the distribution of benefits and burdens, advantages and disadvantages in any given society.

Moreover, in some cases they intersect, leading to a compounding effect on those groups existing at the intersections of these oppressions. One way these processes of social exclusion express themselves is through the differential experience of poverty, hence the feminization and racialization of poverty. I briefly explore that experience and the extent to which it is implicated in health disparities among populations. Ultimately, I argue for a restructuring of these key institutional arrangements so that, regardless of identity, origins or geography, individuals and groups in society can be actively supported with a healthy environment and right to life and well-being.

Social Determinants of Health and Social Exclusion

The social determinants of health (SDH) approach represents a shift from reliance on lifestyle choices (smoking, diet, exercise, etc.) as the most important predictors of the health status of individuals and populations to acknowledging social and economic characteristics of individuals and populations as essential to explaining and predicting health outcomes (CIHI, 2008). It has now been well established that poor social and economic conditions and inequalities in access to resources and services affect an individual or group's health and well-being, perhaps more so than their "health behaviours." Social factors and social forces determine the health outcomes of individuals and populations. However, this neo-materialist approach to SDH does not fully appreciate the extent to which particular groups in society are shut out of the social, economic, cultural and political systems that determine access to society's resources, nor the effect this has on health outcomes. Increasingly, research shows that conditions arising from various forms of marginalization not only compromise the promise of equal citizenship, but also undermine the well-being of affected individuals and groups in society. The relative social distance that emerges out of the processes of colonization, racialization and feminization of key social arrangements is a product of, and reproduces, social disparities that translate into health disparities. The most important consequences of health disparities are avoidable death, disease, disability, distress and discomfort. Health disparities cost individuals, communities, the health system and Canadian society as a whole (Health Disparities Task Group of the Federal/Provincial/Territorial Advisory Committee on Population Health and Health Security, 2004). Health disparities are inconsistent with Canadian values of equality. They threaten the social cohesiveness of community and society, and they challenge the sustainability of the health system and they undermine the Canadian economy (Wilkinson, 1996; Dugger, 1998; Niggle, 1998; McDonald & Quell, 2008).

Defining Social Exclusion

Broadly defined, social exclusion describes both the structures and the dynamic processes of inequality among groups in society which, over time, structure access to critical resources that determine the quality of membership in society and ultimately produce and reproduce a complex of unequal outcomes (White, 1998). In that regard, social exclusion is both process and outcome. In industrialized societies, social exclusion can be said to be a byproduct of unbridled forms of accumulation whose processes commodify social relations and validate and intensify inequality along racial and gender lines (Byrne, 1999). It is manifest through historical processes of oppression that generate material conditions of economic exclusion and social deprivation and also sociopsychological outcomes that impact the health of affected groups. In Canada such groups include Aboriginal peoples, people with disabilities, immigrants and refugees, racialized groups, single parents, children and youth in disadvantaged circumstances, women, the elderly, gays, lesbians, bisexuals and transgendered and transsexual people (Hyman, 2007; Public Health Agency of Canada, 2008a). Further, it is now well documented that adverse socioeconomic conditions in early life lead to increased health risks in adulthood, thereby creating intergenerational health disparities (UNICEF, 2007).

White (1998) refers to four aspects of social exclusion. The first is exclusion from civil society through legal sanction or other institutional mechanisms. This concept may include substantive disconnection from civil society and political participation because of material and social isolation, created through systemic forms of discrimination based on race, ethnicity, gender, disability, sexual orientation and religion. In the post-September 11 era, racial profiling and new notions of national security seem to have exacerbated the experience of this form of social exclusion. Second, social exclusion refers to society's denial of, or exclusion from, social goods to particular groups. This represents the failure to provide for the needs of particular groups, such as accommodation for persons with disabilities, provision of language services for those whose first language is not English, ensuring income and housing security for the homeless, and enforcing sanctions to deter discrimination and abuse. The third aspect is exclusion from social production, a denial of opportunity to contribute to or participate actively in society's social or cultural activities. And the fourth is economic exclusion from social consumption — meaning unequal access to normal forms of livelihood and differential economic or labour market participation (Innocenti Research Centre, 2007; White, 1998).

Social exclusion assumes a community or a society from which the process of exclusion is affected. The multiple dimensions of exclusion may suggest different ways of drawing the boundaries, and here the discourse on citizenship is helpful in laying claim to the community. The notion of citizenship invokes the state as guarantor of the principle of equality among members. These concepts are time and space specific. In industrialized capitalist societies, social exclusion is largely a byproduct of processes of production, wealth accumulation and consumption that tend to validate particular power relations and persistent forms of oppression and social inequalities. The over reliance on market-based mechanisms for resource and income distribution is compounded by the persistence of patriarchal, colonial and racialized ordering of social arrangements, leading to the institutionalization of systems that privilege men, non-Aboriginal and non-racialized Canadians and disadvantage women, Aboriginal peoples and racialized peoples, economically and socially. This ordering results in differential impacts in living conditions and health outcomes (Galabuzi, 2006; Veenstra, 2009).

Social exclusion is a phenomenon experienced by individuals and communities — communities of common bond and geographical communities. The characteristics of social exclusion tend to occur in multiple dimensions and are often mutually reinforcing. Groups living in low income areas are likely to also experience inequality in access to employment, substandard housing, insecurity, stigmatization, institutional breakdown, social service deficits, spatial isolation, disconnection from civil society, gender and racial discrimination and higher health risks.

These processes are dynamic and, given unequal social and power relations in societies, various social forces engage in struggles to gain better access for certain categories of citizen on the one hand, and to transform oppressive structures, institutional practices and the boundaries of access on the other. So the boundaries of social exclusion vary from society to society, as well as over time within a given society (Jenson & Papillon, 2001). The state, as the central institution through which the solidarity of citizenship is expressed, plays an essential role in determining the boundaries of belonging and the creation of political identities, based on the distinction between members and non-members. This common identity then becomes the basis for maintaining social solidarity despite important cultural, economic and social differences among people with often competing interests.

Dimensions of Exclusion

In Canada as elsewhere, social exclusion is an expression of unequal relations of power among groups in society responsible for determining access to economic, social, political and cultural resources. The assertion of certain forms of economic, political, social and cultural privilege occurs at the expense of those lower in the hierarchy of power. This is especially true in a neoliberal market regulated society, where the impetus for state intervention to reduce the reproduction of inequality is minimal. Social exclusion has time and spatial dimensions, suggesting that it emerges out of dynamic processes of oppression. Key aspects of social exclusion are manifested in the economy, in living conditions and in the experience with poverty, but also in contact with key institutions in society such as the criminal justice system, the health care system, the education system, neighbourhood selection and in access to political processes. All of these have implications for the health status of affected groups.

In everyday life, social exclusion defines the inability of particularly affected groups to participate fully in Canadian life due to structural inequalities in access to social, economic, political and cultural resources arising out of the often intersecting experiences of oppression relating to race, class, gender, disability, sexual difference, immigrant status and so on. Along with the socioeconomic and political inequalities, social exclusion is also characterized by processes of group or individual isolation within and from key Canadian societal institutions, such as the economy, the school system, the criminal justice system and the health care system, among others. These engender experiences of social and economic vulnerability, powerlessness, voicelessness, a lack of recognition and sense of belonging, limited options, diminished life chances, despair, opting out, suicidal tendencies and increasingly, community or neighbourhood violence. In addition to numerous adverse health implications, institutional breakdown, community distress and precariousness in living conditions represent a threat to social cohesion and economic prosperity. These threats are characterized by phenomena such as resorting to the informal economy and community violence. There is a need to interrogate the multiple dimensions of the phenomena as well as to identify the subgroup dimension of the victims of social exclusion, precisely because of the extent to which their experiences are differentiated by the nature of the oppressions they suffer. However, there are also points of convergence that define intersectional identities and experiences of oppression. These points can be the basis for solidarity and common struggles against marginalization.

Economic Exclusion
Attachment to the labour market is central to full membership in any society and, in a capitalist liberal democratic society, it is the foundation of full citizenship. It represents a source of livelihood as well as a means for identity formation, and provides a sense of belonging. Attachment to the labour market is particularly central to redressing all forms of exclusion, whether that be reconciling marginalized groups to society or integrating immigrants into the host society — challenges that increasingly face us in Canada. Research on income disparities arising from uneven attachment to labour markets shows that these have adverse impacts on a range of social indicators of well-being, including health status, housing status, educational attainment and political participation, to name a few.

Two key processes underway in Canadian society have made poverty among historically oppressed groups an increasing source of concern. One is the changing economy under the assault of neoliberal restructuring, which has imposed new vulnerabilities on working populations just as precariousness has become more prevalent in the labour market. This is largely because neoliberal restructuring and demands for flexibility have made precarious employment the fastest growing form of work — hence the prevalence of irregular work arrangements and non-standard contracts, temporary, part-time, piece and shift work, and self-employment — coupled with job insecurity, poorer working conditions and loss of control over workplace decision-making (Saunders, 2003; Vosko, 2006). The other process is the persistence of racial and gender hierarchies in the distribution of opportunities in the labour market. The compound effect is that these processes have intensified the impact of social exclusion in the last two decades under the neoliberal regime.

While these developments have placed all workers in a vulnerable position, these vulnerabilities are unevenly distributed because of the pre-existing gendered and racialized hierarchies that produce greater adverse impacts for women, persons with disabilities, Aboriginal peoples, racialized workers and new immigrants. In other words, the impacts of flexible deployment of labour and the attendant insecurity have combined with historical processes of discrimination in employment to impose added vulnerabilities on women, Aboriginal peoples and racialized groups in the Canadian economy (Galabuzi, 2004b). As a consequence of their vulnerability, these groups are exposed disproportionately to the adversities of precarious work. Research shows that this translates into disproportionate exposure to lower incomes and occupational status in comparison to other Canadians.

Poverty and Oppression as Mutually Constitutive Determinants of Health

International and Canadian research has established connections between economic status and the life chances of groups and communities. The WHO (2008a) has reported clearly that the state of economic development is a strong determinant of the health situation of a country. The same goes for inequality in socioeconomic status — the scale of social and economic differences among groups in the population. The more equal the society is, the healthier it is. Social inequality translates into health inequality. Health disparities suggest to us that there are differential experiences in the quality of life enjoyed by different groups in society.

Research shows that poverty is related to higher risks of a whole range of health conditions as well as unhealthy lifestyle choices. Poverty is now widely understood as a social determinant of health (WHO, 2008a). This suggests

102

that social and economic conditions and inequalities in access to resources and services may have a greater impact on an individual or group's health and well-being than their behaviours. Therefore, groups experiencing low income tend to sustain higher health risks and lower health status. Because health inequity is closely linked to socioeconomic inequality, it is important to explore how poverty affects particular populations in society and the implications of that experience for health status.

Poverty is an experience driven by processes of social, political and economic deprivation whose outcomes lead to social exclusion. Poverty in Canada is linked to changes in the economy that have led to the concentration of wealth and economic power in the hands of a few and a growing inequality in incomes. Poverty persists because it is a structural problem due to institutional arrangements to distribute resources, not individual's character flaws. It is connected to how access to opportunities is distributed and efforts rewarded, including the distribution of benefits and burdens, as well as advantages and disadvantages in the labour market. The reality is that many people are adversely affected by the growing polarization in income and wealth and the loss of meaningful social and economic opportunities in the midst of this supposed plenty. The growth in precarious employment — part-time, temporary, contract, work — means more people are job-insecure and vulnerable to being poor, and a disproportionate number of these people are racialized and women.

While the current deepening polarization in income and wealth can be traced to economic restructuring during the last quarter century and state deregulation that enables the market to dictate how the economy should be organized, the persistence of poverty has its roots in the structures and hierarchies of class, race, gender and disability, which determine who the winners and losers are in Canadian society. This process means that these trends are not just passing concerns. Rather, they are enduring because the structures that create inequality are built into the very foundation of society and the economy. Canada was founded as a settler capitalist colony that required the subordination of Indigenous people and their way of life and economy so that their resources could be harnessed for the capitalist machine, first in Europe and then domestically.

From its early days, the Canadian state created institutions that operated in a way that economically, socially and politically disadvantaged some people along lines of class, gender, race, disability and sexual difference, among others. These determine the life chances, quality of education, access to society's resources, where one lives and how one participates in society. These different forms of exclusion are hierarchical and often intersecting in the way they determine the experience of individuals and communities in Canada. The Canadian experience suggests that structural inequality is both gendered and racialized, with the compounded experience leading to deep experiences of social exclusion. The fact that they exist at an intersection of oppression may explain why racialized women are particularly vulnerable to poverty.

Within the context of social exclusion as a relational process, poverty is also a social relational phenomenon encompassing social and economic deprivation. Differential control over access to resources and outcomes, such as the inability to satisfy basic needs, inadequate shelter, poor health, malnutrition, unequal access to public goods (such as transportation, recreation, social services, education and skills training) also intensifies vulnerability to shocks, violence and crime, lack of political participation and voicelessness in society. It is therefore multidimensional in its impact and expression. However, poverty is also differentially experienced by particular groups in society depending on their vulnerability. These vulnerabilities arise from the oppressions these groups face. For example, colonization, structural racism or patriarchy define access to processes of production and to society's resources and lead to differential exposures to low income.

To better understand the intersection between poverty, health and oppression, we need to pay close attention to the factors that contribute to the weakness in the livelihood base and security of those living in poverty. We particularly need to address the bases or sources of vulnerability responsible for the disproportionate exposure to poverty for particular groups such as women, and even more particularly, single mothers, Aboriginal peoples and the colonial relations that define their experience in Canadian society, persons with disability, racialized peoples and especially those who live at the intersections of these bases of oppression. Colonialism, racism, sexism and ableism are all key considerations in that they compound the vulnerabilities that communities experience in an economy that is already unequal in the way it distributes opportunities and outcomes.

For the purposes of understanding existing poverty, it is important to address the specific characteristics of those who experience it. Different groups in society experience poverty differently, some more profoundly than others. For instance, in Canada there are high levels of child poverty and women living in poverty. Average poverty among seniors has declined, though not for all seniors. We have disproportionately more poor among Aboriginal people, women, racialized groups and persons with disability, to name but a few identifiable groups that experience poverty differently. These differences arise from the different oppressions that structure the lives of different groups in society.

In a capitalist society, the poverty generating structures and processes that systematically create winners and losers are compounded by the racial and gendered hierarchies that structure distinctive experiences of inequality for various groups in society. We now know that poverty and social inequality breed alienation and marginalization, and ultimately social strife, social instability, unrest and often violence. As racial and gender hierarchies generate inequality in society and poverty in communities, they become even more entrenched, transforming communities into deep marginalization and exclusion. The compounded effect creates a real threat to social cohesion, often provoking securitized responses that inevitably focus on the marginalized "other" as a threat to society. These manifestations of social exclusion not only represent a threat to the very social fabric of society but to the well-being of its members.

Poverty as a process of marginalization and social exclusion impacts the health status of affected groups. The feminization and racialization of poverty compound racial and gender generated inequalities in material conditions in socially excluded communities. The racialization and feminization of poverty here refers to the disproportionate and persistent incidence of low income among racialized groups and women in Canada. Documented characteristics of the feminization and racialization of poverty (e.g., labour market segregation and low occupation status; high and frequent unemployment status; substandard housing in distressed neighbourhoods; homelessness; poor working conditions; the intensification of work through extended hours of work or multiple jobs; experience with everyday forms of racism and sexism) lead to unequal health service utilization and differential health status.

For example, national and metropolitan area data show that racialized groups experience deepening levels of poverty three times higher than the corresponding averages (Hou & Picot, 2003a). Recent work focusing on neighbourhood analysis of low income in Ontario shows that in 2006, racialized groups made up 45.8 percent of the population living in major urban centres where the poverty rate is 25 percent or greater, an increase from 39.4 percent from 2001. In Toronto, the proportion is as high as 59 percent. The proportion of racialized groups living in low-income areas in the Toronto Census Metropolitan Area in 2006 was 35 percent, compared to 19 percent for non-racialized groups. Rates varied to as high as 50 percent for Africans, 41 percent for West Asians, 40 percent for all Blacks, 39 percent for Latin Americans, 37 percent for Chinese and South East Asians and 31 percent for South Asians (Statistics Canada, 2006d). According to the Toronto Public Health report titled: *The Unequal City: Income and Health Inequalities in Toronto — 2008*, 76 percent of Toronto children living in low-income households are racialized (McKeown, MacCon, Day, et al. 2008).

Racial and Gendered Implications of Social Exclusion for Health Outcomes

Canada's universal health care system has been hailed as a core value of Canadian identity and citizenship. However, this commitment to equal access to health care services is undermined by the documented persistence of health disparities among specific identifiable groups. There is a gap between the promise of universal health care and the differential health status arising from inequalities in the social determinants of health. According to the Health Disparities Task Group (2004), these disparities are discernable based on key characteristics such as socioeconomic status (SES), Aboriginal and other racial identity, gender status and geographic location (pertaining to neighbourhood selection). These key factors associated with health disparities in Canada impose differential costs on individuals and communities as they interact with the health system and lead to differential health outcomes for communities (Agnew, 2002; Anderson, 2000; Health Canada, 2003).

From a social determinants of health perspective, a synthesis of a diverse public health and social scientific literature suggests that the most important antecedents of human health status are not medical care inputs or health behaviours, such as smoking, diet and exercise, but rather social and economic characteristics of individuals and populations. For socially excluded groups, power relations, identity and status issues, and life chances are influential factors when it comes to well-being and health outcomes. Social exclusion influences health through differential exposure to determinants of health by restricting socioeconomic mobility and differential access to resources, even as oppression-related effects such as trauma, stress reactions and depressed self-esteem negatively impact health outcomes (Brondolo, ver Halen, Pencille, et al., 2009).

Research indicates that individuals living in households with incomes below $20,000 are almost three times more likely to experience a decline in self-rated health than people with the highest incomes (Orpana, Lemyre, & Gravel, 2007). Research from multiple sources has shown that low income Canadians have the highest mortality rates, the lowest life expectancy rates and the highest rates of hospitalization and emergency visits. Infant mortality rates have been declining overall, but the rates in the poorest neighbourhoods remain two-thirds higher than in the richest, and the gaps have not closed since 1996. Poverty rates and child poverty rates are disproportionately high among racialized Canadians. Approximately 52 percent of low-income children in Canada live in female-led, single-parent families, according to Campaign 2000, while 49 percent of children in immigrant families and 34 percent of children in racialized families are poor (Campaign 2000, 2008). In fact, according to Lightman, Mitchell, and Wilson (2008), if the incomes of those with the lowest 20 percent of income were raised to the second quintile, the 20 percent to 40 percent level, there would be health related savings of $7.6 billion a year (Spence, 2008). Another way of looking at it is that for every $1,000 in additional income for the poorest 20 percent of Canadians, there would be nearly 10,000 fewer chronic conditions, and 6,600 fewer disability days lost every two weeks (Lightman, Mitchell, & Wilson, 2008). Only 47 percent of Canadians in the bottom income quintile report their health as excellent or very good, compared with 73 percent in the top quintile. People in the lowest quintile are five times more likely to rate their health as fair or poor than people in the highest. Female-led, single-parent families face the highest level of poverty in Canada, with 35 percent living below the poverty line (Spence, 2008).

In relation to oppressions arising from colonization, Aboriginal people experience persistent income inequalities and health inequities, which are exacerbated by colonial relations and structural racism in Canada (Sterritt, 2007). Aboriginal people have lower levels of self-rated health than the total Canadian population. They are twice as likely to report fair or poor health status than non-Aboriginal peoples with the same income levels (Health Canada, 2003). The death rate from injury among Aboriginal infants is four times the rate for Canada as a whole and three times among teenagers. It is estimated that one in every two Aboriginal children live below the poverty line (Bennett & Blackstock, 2007). Aboriginal people have lower life expectancy than other Canadians, with the Inuit having the lowest life expectancy of Aboriginal peoples — twelve years less than the Canadian average. In fact, the life expectancy gap is widening, not decreasing for the Inuit (Statistics Canada, 2006b). Between 2002 and 2006, the tuberculosis rate among the Inuit was ninety times higher than in the non-Aboriginal population in Canada (Minsky, 2009). Aboriginal people are two to three times more likely to develop Type 2 diabetes than the general population (Minsky, 2009).

In 2009, UNICEF described the health disparities facing First Nations, Inuit and Métis children as one of the most significant children's rights challenges facing our nation (UNICEF, 2009). Soroka, Johnson and Banting (2007) have highlighted the persistent inequity in health of Aboriginal people and commented that the lack of belonging, power, participation and empowerment of Aboriginal people is a great challenge to social cohesion in Canada. Studies also show that Aboriginal youth suicide increases in communities where there is a lack of cultural continuity, power, social participation and empowerment (Arundel & Associates, 2009; WHO, 2008a).

Racial oppression may help explain why in Ontario, South Asians and Blacks have the highest levels of hypertension (30 percent and 31 percent, respectively), compared to 21 percent in the general population. Blacks also develop hypertension at earlier ages, with nearly 50 percent developing hypertension in their forties and fifties (Leenen, Dumais, McInnis, et al.,

2008). While there are limited specific data on diseases in Canada relating to racialization, there are indications that the onset of diabetes ranges from 37 percent among recent immigrants to 51 percent among longer term residents in South Asian and Chinese immigrant communities (Spitzer, 2007a). Young Blacks are four times (10.1 per 100,000) as likely to be victims of gun-related homicides as other members of the population (2.4 per 100,000) (Gartner & Thompson, 2004).

Gender is known to shape the distribution of resources and opportunities, power relations, perceptions of capacities and ways of knowing. It is an important determinant of health, and gender oppression is related to the health status of women (Anderson, 2000). The Canadian Women's Health Surveillance Report examines data about the health of Canadian women with a focus on determinants of health that are more prominent for women than men, for example, multiple role strain and the burdens associated with caregiving (CIHI, 2006). Multiple and intersecting stressors for immigrant women have been described as well, including poverty, gender discrimination, low social status, social injustice, losses of social support, family issues and changes in marital relationships (Ahmad, Shik, Vanza, et. al., 2004; Meadows, Thurston, & Melton, 2001).

Research shows that the actual experience of inequality, the impact of relative social deprivation and the stress associated with it tend to have pronounced psychological effects and to impact health status negatively. Race, gender, disability and immigration status are social determinants of health from both a socioeconomic and a sociopsychological perspective (Ahmed, Mohammed, & Williams, 2007; Harrell, Hall, & Taliaferro, 2003). Along with the negative health effects of social and material deprivation, social exclusion and the stress of dealing with it have psychological effects that impact negatively on health status (Kawachi, Kennedy, & Wilkinson, 2000). Social exclusion impacts self-esteem and mastery (perceived control over one's circumstances), which in turn affects the physical and mental health of excluded groups. Processes of marginalization, disempowerment and social exclusion help explain why immigrant health deteriorates over time in the United States and Canada (Viruell-Fuentes, 2007; Grove & Zwi, 2006). The sociopsychological dimension speaks to the historical and persistent modes of marginalization related to racism, sexism and other oppressions in their everyday form. They have particular adverse impacts on health, especially mental health. The impact of colonial relations, the legacy of slavery, the persistence of structural racism and patriarchy as political, economic and cultural forces that organize the everyday lived experiences of socially excluded group members account for the real and perceived vulnerabilities in health status. For instance, racism is a primary source of traumas and other distresses, macro and micro stressors that exacerbate such conditions as mood disorders, hypertension and drug and substance use, in racialized group communities.

In the American context, Dr. Camara Jones (2002: 56) notes: "Black folks are at a higher risk of hypertension, but in childhood, there are no differences between Blacks' and Whites' blood pressure rates.... By the time you get into 24–44 year old groups, you start to see the changes. Her work presents evidence that among White people, blood pressure is dropping at night, but not in Black people." She attributes this to the stress generated by the experiences of everyday racism — having to fend off the causal diminution, put downs and denials of opportunity. Her research found that 22 percent of Blacks surveyed constantly think about their race, while 50 percent do so at least once a day. Among Whites, there was no noticeable preoccupation with their race. Among immigrants, state-imposed barriers to family reunification through immigration policies that discourage it in favour of independent class immigration, lead to extended periods of family separation. Family separation and failure to effect reunification robs family members of their support network but also engenders separation anxiety, thoughts of suicide, lack of sufficient support mechanisms and even death (Dunn & Dyck, 1998). For many racialized groups, racism as a stress generator is compounded by family separation through immigration, the intensification of work, devaluation and worth through decredentialism, and the very experience of inequality and injustice. Stress, in turn, is a major cause of a variety of health problems, particularly mental health. In fact, a Canadian mental health report suggested a connection between mental health and social issues such as racism and discrimination (Government of Canada, 2006). The compound effect of experiences of racism and discrimination has been identified as one of the reasons the health status of racialized populations and immigrants declines over time (Takeuchi & Williams, 2003).

While Canadian literature in this area is somewhat underdeveloped, there is substantial research and literature in the United States suggesting that there is special relevance to looking at racial differences in mental health status (Fernando, 2003). We need to consider closing the knowledge gap by undertaking similar work in the Canadian context (McGibbon & Etowa, 2009).

Spatial Dimensions of Social Exclusion and Health

It is generally accepted that low-income geographical communities sustain higher health risks. Research shows that residents of low-income neighbourhoods have poorer physical and mental health than residents of high-income neighbourhoods (Ross & Mirowsky, 2001; Lemstra, Neudorf, & Opondo, 2006; Truong & Ma, 2006). Racial and gender hierarchies play a role in structuring these health disparities. According to Abada, Hou and Ram (2007), racialized youth living in Canadian neighbourhoods with a high concentration of racialized groups were more likely to report poor health and depression than their counterparts in White neighbourhoods. In Toronto, studies show that low-income neighbourhoods with a high percentage of residents of immigrant and racialized status had higher diabetes rates than higher income neighbourhoods clustered in the centre of the city (Glazier & Booth, 2007).

Social exclusion also takes on a spatial dimension in that particular groups tend to be concentrated in specific areas where living conditions contribute to their marginalization and to higher health risks. In the United States, such concentrations occur in what are termed the "inner cities." In the Canadian context, although there is a limited history of inner-city, in low income neighbourhoods, some highly racialized, patterns are largely different (Schultz, Williams, Isreal, et al., 2002). Lovell (2009) suggests that poverty, race and gender are critical factors in urban health and co-determine health outcomes in urban Canada. The high rates of unemployment and precarious forms of employment, inadequate housing, low income, and single-parents all contribute to high health risks in urban centres, as do the concentrations of racialized and immigrant populations, faced with issues of adequacy, suitability and affordability in access to housing, and the emergence of the "ethnic enclaves" (Census Tracts with at least 30 percent of the population being from a single visible minority group) (Hou & Picott, 2003b).

Inner-city residents face health risks associated with pollutants, HIV infections, tuberculosis, diabetes, drugs and so on. These risks often arise from vulnerable access to economic, political and social power, as well as experiences of oppression relating to class, race and gender, to name a few (Wasylenki, 2001). There is an historical pattern to these experiences. Residential segregation has often shaped the distribution of racialized and non-racialized people in urban centres. At the turn of the last century, Montreal contained what were referred to as "Black districts," where the mortality rate was three times as high as elsewhere in the city. In Hamilton, Ontario, the inner city is dominated by disproportionate numbers of racialized and low-income residents at greater risk of air pollution and such related ailments as heart and lung diseases. Moreover, the social exclusionary experiences of many of these residents means that they are more likely to be unaware of the health risks or ignore them for employment and housing affordability reasons. Winnipeg's North End was defined by its low-income Aboriginal neighbourhoods, as was Vancouver's East End and Calgary's East End, which represent a mixture of racialized immigrant and low-income communities with high levels of single parents who are largely women. In fact, according to Lovell (2009), between 1970 and 1985, there was a widening gap between the incomes and deprivation levels of inner city residents and suburban dwellers in Montreal, Ottawa-Hull, Hamilton, Halifax and Victoria. However, it is increasingly the inner suburbs that contain pockets of low income that intersect with disproportionate levels of single-parent families and racialized and immigrant people (Hulchanski, 2007). This is partly because inner-city suburbs were largely sites for public housing developments and major high-rise rental communities during the postwar Keynesian welfare state economic expansion. It is in these neighbourhoods that low- to middle-income communities settled and that are available to low-income and immigrant populations in the late twentieth and early twenty-first century.

Racialization of poverty in Calgary is a growing phenomenon, with racialized groups a growing segment of the poor in the city — comprising 30 percent in 1996 and rising to 40 percent in 2006 (Pruegger, 2009). The city is also seeing an increasing geographic concentration of racialized poverty, with more than thirty communities where between 60 and 80 percent of the low-income population is racialized and seven communities in which over 80 percent of the low-income population is racialized (Pruegger, 2009). Moreover, according to Pruegger's study, a high number of the racialized population, particularly youth, feel alienated from society and indicate that they face racism and discrimination in everyday life. There are growing concerns that as immigration escalates in the "New West," particularly with the expanded use of the Temporary Foreign Worker Program (TFWP) by employers, the city is creating an underclass of low-skilled, racialized workers, many of whom are subject to exploitation and a segregated labour market (Byl, 2009). These conditions are increasingly typical of urban Canada and have implications for individual and group health. According to the Toronto Public Health report mentioned earlier (2008), low-income and disadvantaged communities have higher rates of illnesses, including diabetes (McKeown, MacCon, Day, et al. 2008). Neighbourhood factors are associated with the risk of diabetes, along with poor diet, lack of physical activity and pollution exposure (Finkelstein, 2008). In Ontario, women living in the lowest income quintile neighbourhoods have 25 percent higher odds of delivering their babies prematurely and 46 percent higher odds of a low-birth-weight baby (Urquia, Frank, Glazier, et al., 2007). Reutter, Steward, Veenstra, et al. (2009) report that the "stigma" of poverty has a negative effect on the physical and mental health status of those living in poverty. According to Warman (2007), what are referred to as ethnic enclaves had a negative impact on the social economic status of immigrant women, particularly those who had most of their education outside Canada.

Neighbourhood selection and residential segregation represent a dimension of social exclusion that expresses itself in community distress and institutional decline, which threaten social cohesion and well-being. According to a report by the Canadian Institute of Well-being, (Scott, 2010), there is an association between an individual's sense of belonging and their general health status. The report suggests a connection between self-rated health and social inclusion, arguing that poorer health is associated with a lack of inclusion. A similar connection has been identified between sense of belonging and mental health. According Shields (2008), about 81 percent of people who said they had excellent or very good mental health reported a strong sense of community belonging, compared to 64 percent who reported a very weak sense of belonging.

Conclusion

I have suggested that social exclusion is both a process and structure of inequality that determines individual and group access to the wealth and resources of society. These processes include various forms of oppressions that impact the conditions of everyday life for particular groups in society. Colonization and racial and patriarchal orders represent hierarchical structures that impose burdens and disadvantages for some groups and secure benefits and privileges for others in society. These processes and structures generate social, economic and political inequalities that lead to differential experiences and outcomes, including health disparities in society. The social determinants of health approach establishes the material and sociopsychological impacts of oppression on health status as manifested in higher rates of unemployment and precarious employment; inadequate, unsuitable and unaffordable housing; low income; unequal access to health services; and increased contact with the criminal justice system.

This chapter discusses three key dimensions of social exclusion relevant to individual and population health — economic exclusion, the racialization and feminization of poverty and the spatial dimension of exclusion. Thus, the most appropriate and effective way to improve overall population health is by addressing the social exclusion of those disproportionately affected by health disparities. That means taking action on the social factors known to influence health. The focus ought to be on the various oppressions that often compound the experience of poverty as a base of disadvantage in society — oppressions relating to race, gender, immigrant status and disability among others. The public health system has an important role to play in mitigating the causes and effects of the social determinants of health through interventions with socially marginalized individuals, populations and communities.

• 8 •

Oppression and Im/migrant Health in Canada

Denise Spitzer

Can migrating make you sick? Most im/migrants[1] enter the country in better health than native-born Canadians in a phenomenon known as the "healthy immigrant effect." In fact cities with a higher percentage of recent immigrants report better than average health status compared to urban centres with fewer foreign-born residents (Gilmore, 2004). Observed in other multi-ethnic, immigrant-receiving countries as well, the healthy immigrant effect refers to the trend wherein the health status of new arrivals, which starts off as superior to that of the local populace, erodes to the point where it converges with and then declines below the general health status of the native-born population (Llácer, Zunzunegui, del Amo, et al., 2007; Ng, Wilkins, Gendron, et al., 2005; Vissandjée, Desmeules, Cao, et al., 2004). This phenomenon is underpinned by the presumption that those who emigrate are in sufficiently good health to make the journey (Ng, Wilkins, Gendron, et al.), and the statistics appear to bear out this assertion. The age-standardized mortality rates for im/migrants are lower than those of their Canadian-born counterparts. The same holds true for refugees — although they perish at higher rates than newcomers who are categorized as voluntary migrants (Hyman, 2007).

Importantly, this deterioration of health status is neither universal nor uniform (Hyman 2007; Llácer, Zunzunegui, del Amo, et al., 2007). Im/migrants from outside Europe (i.e., persons of colour) are twice as likely to experience a deterioration in their health than European-Canadians (Ng, Wilkins, Gendron, et al, 2005). However, higher income appears to mitigate the decline as does having a partner — or at least "somebody to make them feel loved" (Dunn & Dyck, 2000, p. 2000). Women, particularly those from non-European countries, again, are most apt to report worsening health status when compared to their Canadian-born counterparts or foreign-born males (Vissandjée, Desmeules, Cao, et al., 2004). The question remains as to why certain groups of newcomers, particularly racialized and female populations, are more apt to report a decline in their health status over time than others.

From a biomedical perspective, disease and the resultant ill health are rooted in a specific, identifiable etiology — one that is uniform, universal and extracted from social or individual context (Raphael, Curry-Stevens, & Bryant, 2008; Singer, 2004). These etiologies range from genetic anomalies and microscopic organisms to injuries and individual health behaviours. Indeed health-related behaviours such as smoking, alcohol intake, physical activity and food habits are regarded as the prime individual, modifiable factors that can lead to a host of identifiable, deleterious outcomes if healthy choices are not made. As discussed in Chapter 2, these behaviours are the primary target of biomedical interventions and health promotion programs. With regards to im/migrants, a common presumption is that new residents alter their diets from what they had at home, consuming more meat and foods with higher fat, sugar and carbohydrate content, thus leading to increased obesity and other conditions related to poor quality nutrition. But can poor health behaviours account for im/migrants' loss of health status?

Ng, Wilkins, Gendron, et al.'s (2005) examination of the National Population Health Survey (NPHS) indicates that not only do newcomers appear to smoke half as much as Canadian-born individuals, they are only slightly more likely to be less physically active than other Canadians. Importantly, the sector of the foreign-born population that appears to be less physically active are recent European im/migrants, precisely the category of newcomers who are least likely to experience worsening health status. While recent non-European im/migrants appear to gain weight in the years soon after their arrival, it is not clear if changes in stature can be attributed solely to changes in diet, or if other factors such as stress or low-income bear as great or even greater responsibility for this trend (Ng, Wilkins, Gendron, et al., 2005).

In this chapter, I argue that we must relinquish the reductionist lens of the medical gaze in favour of a more complex consideration of im/migrant health that can be situated within a dynamic social context that attends to the social environment, the political economy of health and the body — in essence, a platform upon which we can examine the impact of marginalization and oppression on well-being. I begin by providing a brief overview of the foreign-born population of Canada, and where many are positioned in the social landscape. I suggest that the current manifestations of gendered and structural racism, reflected in increased demands for temporary labour paired with stricter regulations for citizenship and evidenced by newcomers' limited access to social determinants of health, flow from a history of exclusionary immigration policies. Once in the country, the derogation of credentials and foreign work experience, along with shifting gendered, familial and communal demands, constrain social mobility, particularly for foreign-born racialized women. I argue that oppressive circumstances effected through structural and gendered racism are implicated in the disparity between newcomers' dreams of a better life and their realities, the realization of which leads to chronic stress, which is manifested in a variety of ways. Lastly, I briefly discuss how im/migrants may mobilize resources to resist forces of oppression.

Im/migrating to Canada

Each year approximately 225,000 newcomers enter Canada — a country where nearly one in five residents is foreign-born and where immigration accounts for approximately 60 percent of its population growth (CIC, 2005; Gold & Desmeules, 2004; Lindsay & Almey, 2006). From the onset of Confederation, Canadian immigration policy has reflected the demands of business interests and has aided in the constitution of the national imaginary, one that was preferably British and decidedly White. These objectives were reflected in both the recruitment of British women to work as nannies to mother households and set an example to the nation and in the exclusionary measures taken against various countries, ethnicities and religions that would have discoloured it (Green & Green, 2004; Jakubowski, 1997; Li, 2001). In the twentieth century alone, a number of examples illustrate serious exclusionary practices resulting from immigration policies. These includie the notorious *Komagata Maru* incident, which brought national attention to the consequences of extraordinary measures taken to exclude South Asian migrants from Canada; restrictions on Chinese immigration, first of women who hoped to join male family members who had built the railroad, and then of men and women; and the denial of entry to Jewish refugees fleeing the impending genocide in Europe when dominant sentiments were summed up by one politician who infamously remarked: "None is too many" (Abella & Troper, 1983; Jakubowski, 1997).

Changes to immigration policies in the late 1960s, created a shift away from primary considerations of country of origin to a focus on skills and education, opening up Canada to newcomers from outside Europe (Green & Green, 2004). The result has been a dramatic shift in the demographic profile of the country, where now nearly 20 percent are foreign-born. At present, China, India and the Philippines comprise the major source countries of immigrants to Canada while Mexico, Haiti and Colombia are the three main sources of refugee claimants (CIC, 2009).

The categories "immigrant" and "refugee" are meant to reflect the relative voluntariness of migration, with immigrants (economic immigrants and their dependents and family class migrants) viewed as being more skilled, educated and prepared for their journey, while refugees are concomitantly constructed as the wretched of the earth, swept up by the forces of politics and history, and/or as untrustworthy narrators exaggerating or misrepresenting circumstances to their benefit (Knudsen, 1995; Valverde & Pratt, 2002). The boundaries between these categories are slippery and represent geopolitical interests that can structure inclusion and exclusion and reinforce them through social and bureaucratic processes. The category under which a person migrates to Canada has considerable impact on their trajectory as a newcomer settling in this country because it determines access to services, credential adjudication, choice of residence, government employment and access to post-secondary education. The categories and their relative status are further reflected in the highly gendered profile of applicants. Between 1994 and 2003, only 11 percent of principal economic class applicants were female (Lindsay & Almey, 2006). Educated women who enter Canada under the auspices of refugee or family class programs are vulnerable to attitudes, policies and procedures that relegate them to the status of an accessory to a skilled or wealthier applicant or as part of the great unwashed, and presumably uneducated, masses (Kofman, 2004; Spitzer, 2011).

In addition to immigrants and refugees, Canada also facilitates the importation of labour through temporary worker programs (TWPs). TWPs, such as the Seasonal Agricultural Worker Program (SAWP), are used to attract and extract labour from individuals who, while contributing to the Canadian economy, are excluded from enjoying social and political benefits (Preibisch, 2005). Some temporary worker programs, such as the Live-In Caregiver Program (LCP), offer the opportunity of permanent settlement in Canada to select participants (Spitzer & Torres, 2008).[2] Historically, country of origin has figured significantly in policies that have enabled temporary workers to transform their immigration status through the promise of permanent residency (PR) status and citizenship. For instance, when foreign domestic workers were being recruited primarily from the Caribbean, stricter regulations discouraged permanent settlement, while these policies became less restrictive as the Philippines came to dominate LCP recruits (Macklin, 1994).

Im/migrant Lives in Canada

Twenty-four percent of immigrant men and 18 percent of immigrant women possess university degrees, exceeding the average of 16 percent in the general Canadian populace (Lindsay & Almey, 2006; Zietsma, 2007). Very recent immigrants are even better educated; in 2006, nearly 32 percent of newcomers had completed undergraduate university education and another 20 percent had earned graduate degrees (Zietsma, 2007). The employment status of new Canadian residents is often not commensurate with their educational background. Indeed foreign-born men are twice as likely — and foreign-born women are three times as likely — to be unemployed in comparison to their Canadian-born counterparts (Zietsma, 2007). Moreover, those with graduate degrees were unemployed at slightly higher rates than those with undergraduate diplomas, who are already unemployed at nearly four times the rate for university-educated Canadians (Zietsma, 2007).

Those who secure employment may find that their education and work experience does not carry the same weight as it did in their homeland. Haan's (2008) examination of the degree of mismatch between education and work requirements has revealed not only high rates of disconnect between educational background and work status among foreign-born workers in Canada but also important gender and place effects. For example, approximately 30 percent of foreign-born Canadians in metropolitan areas, as compared to just over 11 percent of Canadian-born individuals, are over-qualified for their work. The median annual income for foreign-born Canadians was $25,500, while for native-born Canadians that amount was $42,200. Outside of large cities, the median income of foreign-born Canadians rises slightly to $27,300, while that of native-born Canadians declines slightly to $40,700. Women experience greater mismatch between their education and work status and are less likely to secure a job than men (Haan, 2008; VanderPlaat, 2007), while immigrants and Canadians of non-European ancestry experience greater mismatch than those of European heritage (Haan, 2008; Spitzer, 2009a). Nearly two-thirds of newcomers from Asia and the Middle East are not employed in work commensurate with their educational and occupational backgrounds, while one-third of migrants from Australia, New Zealand and the United States are in similar circumstances (Chui, 2003). These disparities between work and education often translate into downward socioeconomic mobility that for racialized, non-European communities can persist through the next generation (Halli & Kazemipur, 2001). Haan (2008) confirms that education-employment mismatch does not appear to improve over time spent in Canada.

Bauder (2003) describes the consequence of education-employment mismatch as brain abuse. In contrast to brain drain, where highly qualified persons are recruited away from their homelands, brain abuse is characterized by the devaluation of foreign credentials — a situation for which most newcomers are wholly unprepared (Bauder, 2003) — and the erosion of their technical and professional abilities in a process known as de-skilling (Alcuitas, Alcuitas-Imperial, Diocsan, et al., 1997). Problems with recognition of foreign credentials operate to exclude potential workers of certain national origins and/or those possessing degrees from educational institutions in certain countries and to include those whose professional/technical images reify a particular, notably White, Canadian image. Many im/migrants fail to reclaim their occupations and inevitably are integrated into what has become a flexible labour force comprised of well-educated individuals who are willing to work for low wages (Bannerji, 2004; Bauder, 2003).

Increasingly Canada is turning to temporary migrant worker programs to expand this flexible labour force, welcoming migrant workers on one hand, while keeping the other hand on the control levers that allow the government to curtail in-migration and/or to proffer citizenship as a "carrot" that only a select few will have the opportunity to win. Belief in the superiority of the

Canadian educational system, the gatekeeping of Canadian professional or-ganizations and distrust of foreign institutions, particularly of non-European origin, contribute to the derogation of foreign credentials. These sentiments are reinforced in both structural and discursive ways.

Structurally, various exclusionary tactics are deployed to maintain the status quo — the taken-for-granted space of White, heterosexual privilege (Anderson & Reimer-Kirkham, 1998; Page & Thomas, 1994). The degraded cultural capital embedded in the origin and status of educational experience is reinforced by stereotypes that are evoked by the sounds of an accent, the sight of particular phenotypic characteristics such as skin colour and hair type, and the unsettling sensation when confronted with an alternative habitus that signals Otherness — a response that Muslim women in Canada who wear hijabs often confront when trying to enter the labour market (VanderPlaat, 2007). This system of exclusion is underpinned by racialized and/or ethni-cized hierarchies where colonial legacies are reinvigorated and deployed in the service of constructing and upholding a particular (read White) version of citizenship and identity (Grosfugel, 2004). Concomitantly, Canada deploys the language of multiculturalism and cultural diversity to portray our society as tolerant and welcoming, yet this discourse belies social inequalities that are evident to many im/migrants in this country.

Im/migrant Health and Well-Being in Canada

As mentioned in the introduction, newcomers to Canada are often in better health than the average Canadian. As they settle in this country, they tend to underutilize formal health care services, citing problems such as long waiting lists for a family physician — a complaint not uncommon amongst Canadian-born as well (Thurston, Meadows, Este, et al., 2006) — and prolonged waits for gender- and/or linguistically matched-health professionals, while experienc-ing culturally or gender-inappropriate services or procedures (VanderPlaat, 2007). Importantly, foreign-born Canadians encounter challenges with bal-ancing workplace and familial demands, especially with reference to taking time off from paid labour to attend to their health, as many are engaged in precarious employment characterized by part-time work, low-wages and few if any benefits (Lewchuk, de Wolff, King, et al., 2003; Neufeld, Harrison, Hughes, et al., 2002; Spitzer, 2000, 2007b).

Access to health care services, however, is but a single component among many that contribute to the health and well-being of a populace. The deter-minants of health, in particular social determinants such as socioeconomic status, gender and environments, figure prominently in the health status of foreign-born Canadians (Dunn & Dyck, 2000). Research suggests that im/migrants from a variety of source countries define health holistically, equating it with fulfilling one's roles and responsibilities, being able to provide mutual aid to other community members and having meaningful remunerative employment that provides for human dignity (Spitzer, 2007b; Stewart, Anderson, Mwakarimba, et al., 2008).

In other words, for many newcomers to Canada, meaningful labour sufficiently remunerative to cover familial household expenses and to share with others in need is both a goal and a definition of well-being. However, statistics revealing high rates of education/occupation mismatch (Haan, 2008), unemployment (Zietsma, 2007) and poverty, particularly for im/migrants from non-European source countries (Halli & Kazemipur, 2001), suggest that for many newcomers the dreams of a better life — often the primary objective of immigration — have not been realized (Alcuitas, Alcuitas-Imperial, Diocsan, et al., 1997; Bannerji, 2004; Danso, 2001; Spitzer, 2009a; Stewart, Anderson, Mwakarimba, et al., 2008). Professional aspirations give way to survival efforts, and often the dreams of re-establishing their careers or of retraining to meet Canadian requirements are relinquished as immediate financial and familial demands take precedence. These trajectories are not uniform but vary as immigration status intersects with gender, socioeconomic class, ethnicity, religious affiliation, racialized status and place, among other factors. For instance, foreign-born Canadians who are identified as members of racialized communities may be particularly burdened by experiences of racism, which can result in increased hypertension, stress and depression (Din-Dzietham, Nembhard, Collins, et al., 2004; Karlsen & Nazroo 2002). Chapter 2 provides a detailed explanation of the ways that these physical and mental health stresses are linked to oppressive social circumstances.

Women im/migrants face additional challenges in their efforts to re-establish their careers as they are often compelled to balance their desires for educational or occupational advancement with their desires to fulfill their gendered, familial responsibilities, in particular around family caregiving (Spitzer, 2005; Spitzer & Torres, 2008; VanderPlaat, 2007). Because care-work is intimately linked to gender and culture and women's role in social and biological reproduction, care-work has become a central part of the gendered performances that are integral to the establishment of ethnic boundaries (Spitzer, 2005). Although the enactment of caregiving responsibilities can be fulfilling, it may also bind women closer to home and limit their opportunities to enter the labour market, to access supportive networks, to upgrade their skills or to learn French or English as a second language (VanderPlaat, 2007). The lack of affordable child care and the paucity of culturally appropriate, accessible home care and auxiliary health services can contribute to women's isolation, which compounded by their dearth of social capital and few opportunities to accrue more, threatens to marginalize women socially and economically (Neufeld, Harrison, Hughes, et al., 2002; VanderPlaat, 2007).

Downward social mobility and the subsequent loss of professional identities are evidence of structural systemic racism (Krieger, 1999). Institutionalized racism "is often evident as inaction in the face of need" (Jones, 2000, p. 1212) and reinforces the status quo through subtle exclusionary measures that structure access to opportunities and social goods. These forces are reinforced through expressions of circulating stereotypes and racist remarks that sharpen and maintain social divisions and unequal power relations. Most commonly, many forms of racism are experienced simultaneously, resulting in what Essed (1991: 50) terms "everyday racism," — "the integration of racism into everyday situations through practices (cognitive and behavioural…) that activate underlying power relations."

Oppression, Health and the Embodiment of Inequality

The impact of social context on the health and well-being of Canadian im/migrants, most specifically the erosion of health status amongst racialized, gendered newcomers, can be conceptualized in a number of ways. First, the population health framework that highlights the determinants of health dominates the policy discourse in Canada despite concerns about its minimal uptake and poor operationalization with regards to programs and policies (Raphael, Curry-Stevens & Bryant, 2008). The social determinants of health highlight the impact of low socioeconomic status, as well as gender and other social markers on the well-being of individuals and communities. For marginalized groups, such as some Canadian newcomers, deprivation that is characterized by limited access to health determinants may be a theme repeated throughout their lives. As such, they are vulnerable to a syndemic (two or more diseases or health conditions in a population) assault from multiple deleterious health effects, potentially attenuated by their interactions with a noxious social environment (Singer & Clair, 2003).

Second, one can focus on the body as site of experience and sensation, and embodiment as the process of taking up the world and interpreting it back to oneself and others in the creation of intersubjectivity (Spitzer, 2009b). The result of living with the impact of forms of gendered racism includes, most poignantly, the recognition of the gap between one's dreams or expectations and one's lived experience. Discrepant expectations can, therefore, conceivably be regarded as a chronic stressor that underpins the loss of the healthy immigrant effect. This disjuncture between one's hopes and dreams and one's reality can be expressed through the body in ways that elude nosological classification — in the form of amorphous pain for instance — but which are understood by sufferers to be grounded in their material and social circumstances (Coker, 2004; Davis, 1997; Spitzer, 2007b). While the body responds to its physical, social and personal environment in ways that can be interpretive and metaphorical, the embodiment of inequalities can be expressed somatically in ways that are more readily awarded a disease label and presented as an individual condition. In previous research, conditions ranging from hypertension to Type 2 diabetes have been associated with social stressors in general, and in particular to the stress associated with discrepant expectations and downward mobility (Dressler, 1991; Krieger, 1999).

Singer (2004: 17) offers the name "oppression illness," to provide a rubric for the "chronic, traumatic effects of experiencing social bigotry over long periods of time (especially during critical development periods of identity formation) combined with the negative emotional effects of internalizing prejudice." The term offers sufficient elasticity to encompass the health effects of material and social deprivation, stigma and social exclusion as expressed through the body as suffering, or through a cluster of signs and symptoms that can be allocated a disease label. Oppression illness clearly situates the etiology of the condition in the social environment and seeks to unmask the social underpinnings of ill health. In this view, poor health behaviours such as smoking or alcohol consumption are regarded as coping strategies, self-medication in response to the toxicity of one's social world. A European study found that women living in poverty were more apt to die from stress-related conditions such as cardiovascular diseases and Type 2 diabetes, while men perished from conditions relating to tobacco and alcohol consumption. This finding suggests that there are gender disparities in coping strategies that have an impact on how bodies respond to material and social deprivation, with women generally repressing emotions and men dulling their sentiments through chemical substances (Benach, Yasui, Borrell, et al., 2001), thus in-dicating once again that attention to gender as it intersects with other social identifiers is crucial to understanding social phenomena.

Resisting Oppression

Situating oppression illness in the social world refutes the reductionist, biomedical approach that focuses on individual culpability for ill health and highlights interventions that can mitigate the impact of this condition within the realm of social relations. For example, social support is widely regarded as essential to health and well-being, yet many newcomers are compelled to regenerate social linkages with others in Canada as social networks be-come fragmented during the process of immigration (Dunn & Dyck 2000; Stewart, Anderson, Mwakarimba, et al., 2008). Re-establishing social ties, and feeling like one can contribute to society, are not only vital to the health and well-being of individuals, but to communities as well. Moreover, the collective action required to combat the epidemic of oppression illness will need the support of community members, academics, health providers and community workers to address the systemic issues that constrain not only the advancement of foreign-born Canadians but also their ability to share their personal and collective resources with Canadian society.

Conclusion

Immigration policy in Canada, which has always balanced humanitarian with business concerns (Green & Green, 2004), has also been informed by racist sentiments that commonly circulate in Canadian society and which are evidenced by exclusionary measures such as withholding the potential for permanent residency or citizenship. While many newcomers confront challenges settling in this country, foreign-born women of colour appear to report the most profound decline in their health status after residing in Canada for more than a decade (Vissandjée, Desmeules, Cao, et al., 2004). Examining this deterioration of health through a social lens leads to a picture of mostly women spiraling downward socioeconomically as their foreign work experience and credentials are granted little value and as caregiving and familial roles often preclude the possibility of investing time and money into their own skills upgrading. As a result, many find themselves years later living in a country where, despite many positive aspects, everyday racism in subtle and blatant forms is still pervasive and where the dreams of the life they wanted for themselves and their family have not been realized. Chronic stress that results from these discrepant expectations is taken up by the body and responded to in gendered ways that can be regarded as the embodiment of inequality, or as oppression illness. Regardless of label, the relationship between ill health and im/migration requires a holistic vision, one that attends to messages of suffering spoken through the body and one that supports the promulgation of community-based collective action to address racism, sexism and the power inequities that they support.

Notes

1. As the boundaries between the categories of immigrant, migrant and refugee that turn on degrees of voluntariness of movement and on intentions of temporary or permanent resettlement are often slippery and permeable, I follow Tastoglou and Dobrowsky by employing the term im/migrant to refer to all forms of permanent or temporary resettlement. The terms immigrant, migrant and refugee will be used where studies have made specific reference to a particular category and where policy ramifications apply.

2. Temporary worker programs include the Seasonal Agricultural Workers Program, the Live-In Caregiver Program and schemes that enable individual employers to hire non-Canadian workers on a temporary basis to carry out work that they cannot find Canadians to undertake. Recent provisions allow for provinces to nominate some temporary workers for permanent residency status. While this provision is meant to attract potential employees, the number of workers who are actually nominated and who are successfully admitted into this country to settle permanently remains low (Byl, 2009).

9

Oppression and Mental Health

Pathologizing the Outcomes of Injustice

Elizabeth A. McGibbon

> Since the issue of repetitive and circular trauma never truly entered into Western perception, as it was never properly analyzed and never understood, no healing modality was designed to assist Aboriginal people to prepare for, or respond to, the demands associated with such a profound social and cultural loss. (Wesley-Esquimaux & Smolewski, 2004, p. 53)

Oppression is inscribed on the bodies, minds and spirits of oppressed peoples, thus creating clear population disparities in physical and mental health and well-being. When people experience the mental stress of racism and the unjust policies that create and sustain poverty, they are impacted persistently over time. Such everyday mental stress, for example, eventually stresses the body's adrenal system to the point where physical symptoms, such as Type 2 diabetes and high blood pressure, occur as a response to adrenal fatigue. Thus, the physical and mental health outcomes of oppression are synergistic.

This chapter focuses on the ways that oppression is intimately linked to mental and spiritual health and well-being in particular — the inscription of suffering on the soul and the psyche. Evidence is presented to support the relationship between mental health and oppression across the lifespan, thus underscoring that mental health struggles such as depression and chronic anxiety are disproportionately experienced by members of oppressed groups. Chapters 6 and 7 also describe the etiology of some of these struggles and their relationship with Indigenous and im/migrant mental health respectively. This chapter revisits the concept of psychiatrization in the context of the shifting engines of medicalization (Conrad, 2005). Although the history and consequences of medicalization have been discussed extensively elsewhere, psychiatrization has not been sufficiently detailed in the context of patholo-gizing the mental health consequences of oppression. The chapter concludes with a discussion of the centrality of intergenerational trauma transmission as a sequela of oppression.

Mental Health Outcomes of
Oppression-Related Spiritual and Psychological Stress

Ultimately, the mental health outcomes of oppression happen in synergy with physical health outcomes. There has been relatively little attention in the literature, however, to the ways that oppressive societal structures are articulated to psychological and physiological health pathways. Although there is a substantive field of knowledge about the impact of stress on the body's adrenal system and the impact of oppression on marginalized and racialized peoples, discussion of the synthesis of these two areas of knowledge is in its relative infancy. The following section builds on work in these areas to provide a critical perspective on oppression-related stress.

Spiritual and psychological stresses are a core aspect of oppression. Chapter 2 describes in detail the relationships among physical and physiological aspects of oppression, Key features of these stresses are reviewed here to underscore this relationship. As Figure 9.1 illustrates, the mental health consequences of oppression have at least two pathways. The more recognized pathway involves chronic mental health problems resulting from persistent spiritual and psychological distress. The less acknowledged pathway involves chronic mental health problems resulting from persistent distress on the adrenal system — the body's stress-handling system. When individuals, families and communities experience chronic poverty, the cumulative stress of worrying about precarious food, shelter and myriad other deprivations leads to chronic anxiety and sometimes depression. The everyday and relentless nature of this kind of worry is difficult to fathom unless you have personal experience of these material struggles. As Willem de Kooning, the Dutch-born American painter, pointed out: "The trouble with being poor is that it takes up all of your time" (Lake, 2010).

The physical stresses of food insecurity, such as inadequate money for food, especially fresh food, and housing insecurity, such as living in damp housing with insufficient heat, happen in tandem with the spiritual and psychological stress of *chronic worry* about food, shelter and heating. These worries, along with the stresses of everyday racism, sexism, misogyny, homophobia and colonialism, have a profound impact on the body's stress-managing systems — the sympathetic adrenal medulla (SAM) and the hypothalamus-pituitary-adrenal cortex (HYPAC), both located near the brain. The SAM-HYPAC system is structured to deal with everyday stresses in addition to more acute stresses. This system successfully regulates our bodies through short-term stressful times and help us maintain overall wellness. The problem arises when long-term, chronic stress eventually overtaxes the SAM-HYPAC system. The system becomes overwhelmed and is unable to maintain physiological balance. The result is adrenal fatigue. Adrenal fatigue causes depression, obesity, hypertension, diabetes, cancer, ulcers, chronic

Figure 9.1 People Under Threat: Health Outcomes of Oppression-Related Stress

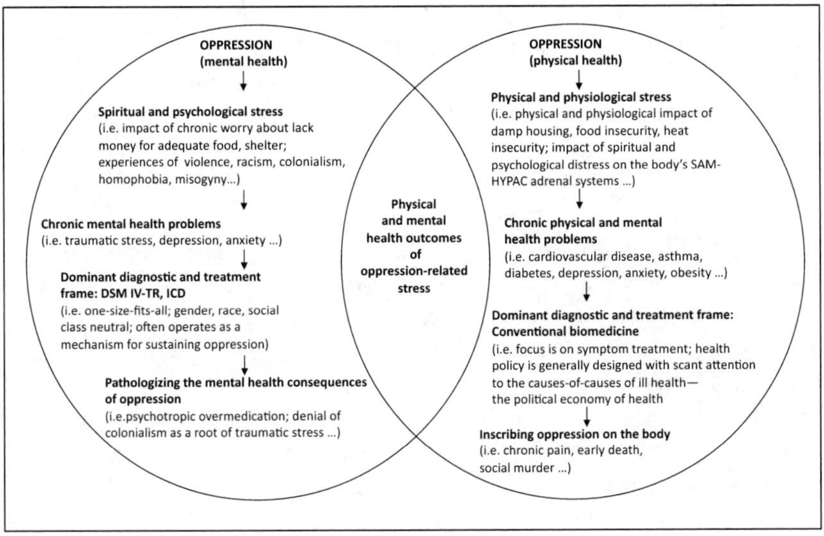

stomach problems, allergies and eczema, autoimmune diseases, headaches, kidney and liver disease and overall reduced immunity (Varcarolis, 2008). These physical and mental health outcomes of adrenal fatigue are embodied in oppressed peoples.

Childhood poverty serves as an urgent example of the chronic stress of oppression. Despite the well-documented links between poverty and child health and despite a unanimous 1989 House of Commons resolution to eliminate child poverty in Canada by the year 2000, the situation has grown progressively worse (McGibbon & McPherson, 2011). More than one million Canadian children, or one child in ten, are still living in poverty — a more than 20 percent increase since 1989 (Campaign 2000, 2009). Furthermore, poverty intersects with racism such that children from racialized groups experience even higher levels of poverty. Social exclusion and the racialization of poverty mean that 51 percent of Canadian Aboriginal children and 42.7 percent of visible minority children in Canada are likely to be poor, compared to the already unacceptable national average of 23.4 percent (CCSD, 2009). Our great national shame is that one in every four children in First Nations communities is growing up in poverty (Campaign 2000, 2009; McPherson & McGibbon, 2010a).

It is also important to note that paid work does not assure a pathway out of family poverty. In the last decade, four in ten low income children had at least one parent who worked full time throughout the year, but who could not rise out of poverty — an increase from less than one out of every three children during the 1990s (Campaign 2000, 2009). Children of recent immigrants, children with a disability, Aboriginal children and children who live in racialized families continue to be among the poorest in the country. In 2005, there were 3.5 million people (10.8 percent of the total population) living on a low income (Statistics Canada, 2006c). These millions of children, adolescents, adults and elders experience the relentless everyday stress of worrying about the basic necessities of life. Oppressions related to social class, gender, race and disability also intersect to create increased poverty (McGibbon & Etowa, 2009).

A key, unique aspect of an environment of poverty is cumulative exposure to multiple adverse physical and social stressors (Evans & English, 2002). Of particular concern is the robust relationship between poverty, or low socioeconomic status, and childhood stress (Evans & Kim, 2007; McPherson & McGibbon, 2010a). This stress causes a wide range of physiological and socio-emotional difficulties in children, including chronic dysregulation of the cardiovascular system, disruption of the body's stress-handling system, described above (Evans & Kim, 2007), depression and low achievement (Alaimo, Olsen, & Frongillo, 2002). The scope and depth of the impact of childhood poverty on long-term mental health is further evidenced by the inverse relationship between poverty and working memory in young adults (Evans & Schamberg, 2009).

Poverty is the strongest determinant of health, regardless of geography. Depression in women and men has been linked to unemployment and adverse working conditions (Bambra & Eikemo, 2008), which are disproportionately experienced by persons in the lower socioeconomic gradients, people of colour and persons with disabilities, regardless of gender (McGibbon, 2009). Social class exploitation sets the stage for, and interacts with, racial discrimination to determine racial inequalities in physical and mental health (Oliver & Muntaner, 2005). Workers in poor families are more likely to lack basic work standards, such as sick leave or time off to care for a sick child. Their jobs are more likely to be unsafe and involve exposure to dangerous substances or working conditions that can lead to economically disruptive injuries and concomitant high levels of stress (Kaplan, 2009). Lone mothers remain the poorest family type in Canada, with a poverty rate (based on a before-tax low income cut-off) of 38.1 percent, compared to 11.9 percent for single fathers (FAIA, 2008). Unattached senior women are also particularly vulnerable to poverty, with 37.2 percent falling below the poverty line, compared to 28.9 percent of unattached older men. Of all senior women, 16.6 percent are poor compared to 8.3 percent of senior men (FAIA, 2008). Poverty rates are 36 percent for Aboriginal women and 29 percent for women of colour. African-Canadian women are the poorest racialized group in Canada, with a poverty rate of 57 percent. The overall poverty rate for foreign-born women is 23 percent, rising to 35 percent for those who arrived between 1991 and 2000 (FAIA, 2008).

People with disabilities are much more likely to experience various forms of material hardship — including food insecurity, not getting needed medical or dental care and not being able to pay rent, mortgage and utility bills — than people without disabilities, even after controlling for income and other characteristics (Fremstad, 2009). Measures of income poverty that fail to take disability into account likely underestimate the income people with disabilities need to meet basic needs (Fremstad, 2009). Violence against people with disabilities has been characterized as occurring in the context of systemic discrimination, and there is often an imbalance of power, including both overt and subtle forms of abuse that may or may not be considered criminal acts (Ticoll, 1994). Twenty-six percent of women with disabilities fall below the poverty line (FAIA, 2008). Almost half of working-age adults who experience income poverty for at least a twelve-month period have one or more disabilities. Nearly two-thirds of working-age adults who experience consistent income poverty — more than thirty-six months of income poverty during a forty-eight-month period — have one or more disabilities. Male household heads reaching their mid-fifties and living in poverty have a 53 percent chance of having been disabled at least once and a 19 percent chance of having a chronic and severe disability (Fremstad, 2009).

Regardless of whether families are living in relative poverty, women and children experience violence in their homes at a disproportionately high rate compared to men. Women around the world, across all age groups, have higher rates of depression than men (WHO, 2000a). Scholars have linked women's depression with unfair distribution of material and financial resources (Belle & Doucet, 2003), family violence and violence due to war and civic unrest (WHO, 2006a). Statistics Canada (2005b) reported that the spousal homicide rate against women was five times higher than the corresponding rate for men. Homicide rates in rural areas were almost identical to rates in urban areas, thus underscoring the comparable vulnerability of rural women. In Canada, spousal violence was the largest category of convictions involving non-specialized adult courts over the five-year period from 1997/98 to 2001/02. Over 90 percent of the offenders were male (Zeitsma, 2006b). Between April 1, 2003, and March 31, 2004, 58,486 women and 36,840 children sought refuge in one of Canada's 473 shelters (Zeitsma, 2006b).

These numbers, and other supporting statistics, led to the moniker "refugee camps" for women's shelters, a term made famous by author Brian Vallee (2007). In *The War on Women*, Vallée revisits the domestic battlefield, revealing that the war on women by the intimate men in their lives continues and that the fallen in this war are more likely to be ignored than honoured. Vallee also points out that the number of men being killed by their spouses has dropped by more than 70 percent since the inception of shelters, while

Table 9.1 Racism: A Social Determinant of Mental Health

Depression
- In the United States, members of racial and ethnic minority groups, including Blacks and Hispanics, are less likely than Whites to obtain treatment for depression (Goldstein, et al., 2006);
- In First Nations adults, 33.4% of women and 28.5% of men report that they have thought about suicide in their lifetime (Assembly of First Nations, 2007).
- In First Nations people between ages 18-34, 21.3% of women and 14.8% of men reported that they attempted suicide in their lifetime (Assembly of First Nations, 2007).
- African-American individuals were substantially more likely to be untreated for depression (37.1%) than Hispanic (23.6%), White (22.4%) or Asian (13.8%) (Strothers, et al., 2005).
- When major depressive disorder affects African Americans and Caribbean Blacks, it is usually untreated and is more severe and disabling compared with that in non-Hispanic Whites (Williams, et al., 2007).

Trauma (Post-Traumatic Stress)
- Post-traumatic stress exists throughout Aboriginal communities in Canada and is a result of the legacy of colonialism and Indian residential schools (Harry, 2008).
- PTSD was found to be a common yet under-recognized and under-treated source of psychiatric morbidity in an urban community of African Americans with low socio-economic status. Despite high rates of trauma/PTSD, this population was not currently identified as being in need of treatment (Schwartz, Bradley, et al., 2005).

Dementia Care
- Even when formal services provide activities of daily living (ADL) care to those with dementia, African American dementia caregivers report more unmet needs with care provision than do White dementia caregivers (Cloutterbuck & Mahoney, 2003)
- Negative, disrespectful health care provider attitudes and behaviour were encountered by African American families during the process of obtaining a diagnosis of dementia for their loved one. They described interactions with health care providers that consistently denigrated, devalued and disrespected their observations and concerns about their demented loved ones. Many reported being shuttled from one health care setting to another in search of a diagnosis (Cloutterbuck & Mahoney, 2003).

Table 9.1 Racism: A Social Determinant of Mental Health

Mental Health –Additional Evidence

- Ethnic minorities with symptoms/histories of mental disorders experience vastly different access and outcome histories when compared to their Caucasian counterparts; ethnic minority people are at risk for not receiving adequate mental health care (Gary, 2005);
- Aboriginal people face racism and discrimination on a day-to-day basis. Cultural discontinuity including loss of Indigenous languages has been associated with higher rates of depression, alcoholism, suicide and violence and as having a greater impact on youth (Health Council of Canada, 2005);
- Among those with perceived need, compared to Whites, African Americans were more likely to have no access to care for alcoholism, drug abuse or mental illness (25.4% versus 12.5%), and Hispanics were more likely to have less care than needed or delayed care (22.7% versus 10.7%). Among those with need, Whites were more likely than Hispanics or African Americans to be receiving active alcoholism, drug abuse or mental health treatment (37.6% versus 22.4%25.0%) (Wells, et al., 2001).
- Disabled Aboriginal seniors are often discriminated against when away from their reserves. To receive needed care, many seniors are forced away from their communities and into unfamiliar, often urban facilities (Kuran, 2002);
- A history of racial discrimination, social exclusion and poverty can combine with mistrust and fear to deter members of racialized groups and Aboriginal communities from accessing services and getting culturally appropriate care (Kafele, 2004).
- Although racialized groups and members of Aboriginal communities have mental health needs and issues that are extremely serious and warrant significant attention, few psychiatric services respond specifically with research, clinical support, programming, organizational change, health promotion or community collaboration that indicate cultural competence, understanding or awareness in a systemic manner (Kafele, 2004).
- Racial profiling, racist assumptions and stereotyping in psychiatry are believed to be strong determining factors in intake, assessment, diagnosis and misdiagnosis. This can account for the non-delivery of appropriate treatments because of an erroneous diagnostic label. Because of disparities and racial discrimination in mental health services, a disproportionate number of racialized groups and Aboriginal populations with mental illnesses do not fully benefit from, or contribute to, the opportunities and prosperity of our society (Kafele, 2004).

*Please note: The information reported in this table cites the terms used by the authors of the articles (i.e., Black, African American, Hispanic, Aboriginal, Ethnic Minority, Visible Minority, White, Caucasian, etc.)

the number of women being killed has dropped by less than 25 percent (Vallee 2007: Abstract).

> From 2000 to the end of 2006, the total of all U.S. military and law enforcement deaths — including accidents and suicides — was 4,588. The combined total of all Canadian military and law enforcement deaths in that period was 101. In that same seven years more than 8,000 women in the U.S. were shot, stabbed, strangled, burned, or beaten to death by the intimate males in their lives. While in Canada, over 500 women — five times more than Canadian soldiers and police officers — were killed by their current or former male partners. Even adding in all the victims of 9/11 to the U.S. law enforcement and military total, it's still less than the number of women killed.

Researchers and others have consistently documented the serious long-term psychological and spiritual impacts of living in an environment of violence, including chronic dysregulation of the adrenal system (Goddard et al., 2010). An estimated 80 percent of 50 million people affected by violent conflicts, civil wars, disasters and displacement are women and children. The World Health Organization (2006) relates the fact that women are the largest single group of people suffering from post-traumatic stress to the high prevalence of sexual violence to which women are subjected.

Racism has consistently been identified as a cause of stress, even when other stress-causing factors are taken into consideration (Pieterse & Carter, 2007), and authors have emphasized the importance of investigating individual, institutional and cultural aspects of racism as forms of stress (Franklin, 2002). Intergenerational stress of the centuries-old legacy of colonization and re-colonization is increasingly documented by scholars and practitioners. Chapters 5 and 7 further explore the mental, spiritual and physical health consequences of racism.

The relationships among oppression and the isms (racism, sexism, classism, heterosexism, ageism, ableism, to name a few) are borne out in an irrefutable body of knowledge about higher anxiety and depression rates among oppressed groups. Research has shown that racial discrimination is associated with depression, thus creating a double jeopardy for persons of colour and triple jeopardy for women of colour (Brown, et al., 2003; Etowa, Keddy, et al., 2007). Off-reserve Aboriginal people were one and a half times more likely than the non-Aboriginal population to experience a major depressive episode in the year before they were surveyed (Statistics Canada, 2002). Young Inuit men have the highest suicide rates in Canada (Statistics Canada, 2003). These examples depict the compounding effects of each oppression. African-American individuals are substantially more likely to be untreated for depression (37.1 percent) than are White individuals. Table 9.1 details more evidence of the differential mental health outcomes associated with the oppression of racism, specifically in the areas of depression, trauma and dementia.

Homophobic discrimination and hatred have a demonstrable and significant impact on the mental health of lesbian, gay, bisexual and transgender (LGBT) people. Mental health struggles in LGBT people are higher than in the general population, and this finding may be related to experiences of social exclusion and discrimination. Between 20 percent and 42 percent of gay and bisexual men have attempted suicide (Douglas Scott, Pringle, & Lumsdaine, 2004). Other health issues identified in research and considered to be fuelled by homophobia include eating disorders, substance abuse, self-harm and alcohol abuse (Douglas Scott, Pringle, & Lumsdaine, 2004). These mental health struggles are universally linked to internalized homophobia and self-hatred, which is, in turn, linked to the discrimination and isolation experienced by people across all ages in LGBT communities.

There is evidence of widespread homophobia amongst doctors and thus a need for increased education about discrimination and LGBT health at medical schools, nursing schools and in the training of other health professions (Douglas Scott, Pringle, & Lumsdaine, 2004). Barriers in access to mental health services for lesbian, gay, bisexual and transgendered adolescents have also been linked to systemic discrimination (McGibbon, 2009). Lesbian, gay and bisexual youth have higher depression and suicide rates than the overall rate for youth (Mederios, et al., 2004; Morrison & L'Heureux, 2001) and are more likely to be homeless than the general youth population (Cochran, et al. 2002).

Pathologizing the Mental Health Consequences of Oppression

Oppressions and their intersections — policy-created poverty, sexism and misogyny, racism, colonialism, and heterosexism, to name a few — create chronic mental health problems, including traumatic stress, depression and anxiety. These struggles are compounded by a mental health system that is grounded in biomedicine and in particular, the field of psychiatry. Along with these mental health problems, intersections of the SDH, the isms and geography, as described in Chapter 2, create barriers in access to mental health care and play an important role in mental health outcomes. As evidenced in this chapter, SDH such as employment, working conditions and housing are strongly associated with an individual's mental health and resiliency. Similarly, gender, race and age (sexism, racism, ageism) are markers of mental health (Ali, Massaquoi, & Brown, 2003; McIntyre, Wien, et al., 2001).

The intersecting relationships among the social determinants of health, the isms and mental health struggles have led to a growing critique of biomedical and in particular, psychiatric approaches to assessment and intervention. An individualistic focus obscures attention to the social and economic conditions that cause or exacerbate mental health problems (McGibbon, 2009). Most publicly funded mental health services in Canada use the psychiatric diagnostic categories outlined in the *Diagnostic and Statistical Manual of Mental Disorders* (DSM-IV-TR) (American Psychiatric Association, 2004). Although the assessment system in the DSM-IV-TR includes a category entitled "psychosocial and environmental problems," its brief (less than two out of 900 pages) description *remained exactly the same* in the 2004 edition as it was in the 1994 edition. Culture, gender and age features are discussed in terms of epidemiological rather than sociological significance (McGibbon, 2009). This token and outdated attention to the influence of the SDH and the isms in the development of mental health and wellness is indicative of a much larger problem in the delivery of mental health services in Canada. Consistent historical reliance on the biomedical model of psychiatry, a framework which has limited capacity for incorporating spiritual, economic and political origins of mental health struggles, has made it next to impossible to develop a mental health system that effectively responds to SDH-related stress (McGibbon, 2009).

In the widely used DSM-IV-TR (2004) classification system, depression is described as a psychiatric disorder. Since experiences of depression and stress are strongly influenced by the SDH, those experiencing stress related to unemployment and adverse working conditions, racism, inadequate or no housing and social exclusion are under threat of the medicalization of problems that are, in fact, structural, systemic problems. Although a critique of biomedical psychiatry has been historically described in detail elsewhere (for example, see Breggin, 2008, 1991; Caplan, 2004; Goffman, 1961; Illich, 1976), it is imperative to underscore the relationship between psychiatrization and oppression. Here, I wish to focus on what Conrad (2005) terms the shifting engines of medicalization and psychiatrization in particular. Medicalization has been defined as the rendering of life experiences as processes of health disorders that can be discussed exclusively in medical terms and to which only medical solutions can be applied (Illich, 1976; Zola, 1978). Behaviours, conditions and experiences are given a medical meaning with narrowly defined parameters and treatments. Psychiatrization is a particular genre of medicalization, and its relationship to the structural determinants of health has received relatively little critical attention within the health fields or even in the social sciences. Although pathologizing the mental health consequences of social injustice has been clearly detailed elsewhere, psychiatrization is not often explicitly identified as a continued mechanism of the apparatus of modern day oppression.

Although many clinicians explore the SDH in the clinical setting, the Canadian diagnostic frame remains rooted in the DSM-IV-TR (American Psychiatric Association, 2004). The international equivalent is the

International Classification of Diseases (ICD-10) (WHO, 2007d). Both of these texts serve as a powerful unifying philosophy that dominates the ways that mental health and illness are framed in the Western world, and increasingly in the Global South. Central to this philosophy are beliefs about the individualistic and apolitical nature of mental illness, the dominance of psychotropic medications as the primary mode of intervention, and the increasing primacy of linkages between the field of psychiatry and the transnational pharmaceutical industry.

The resulting medicalization of oppression causes systemically created social problems to be reframed as individual psychiatric disorders, where clinical treatment continues to heavily rely on psychopharmaceuticals. The efficacy of some psychotropic drugs notwithstanding, stress and anxiety related to oppressive living conditions cannot be ameliorated with pills. For example, recovery from the intergenerational trauma of colonialism, further taken up later in this chapter, requires a much deeper and more sophisticated approach, an approach that the current psychiatric system is ill-equipped to undertake. The above statistics about mental health outcomes provide compelling evidence of injustice and how it becomes embedded in the spirit and the psyche. These are the mental health consequences of oppression, and they have their origins in the structural determinants of health. Although people can and do develop mental health problems that are not rooted in oppression, it is imperative that policymakers, researchers, practitioners and the general public recognize the disproportionate incidence of mental health struggles in those who experience discrimination and oppression.

In order to move forward, it is necessary to tackle the shifting engines of medicalization, once largely confined to the realm of the medical practitioner. Economic globalization has significantly altered the ways that health is conceived and the ways that the market heavily influences the central drivers of the health system. According to Conrad (2005), the ideological centre of medicalization remains constant; however, the engines that drive the medicalization process have shifted. He describes major changes in medical knowledge and organization — including biotechnology, especially the pharmaceutical industry and genetics, and managed care — and how they heavily influence new genres of medicalization.

> Doctors are still gatekeepers for medical treatment, but their role has become more subordinate in the expansion or contraction of medicalization. Medicalization is now more driven by commercial and market interests than by professional claims-makers. The definitional center of medicalization remains constant, but the availability of new pharmaceutical and potential genetic treatments are increasingly drivers for new medical categories. (Abstract)

These changes, especially the emergence of the biotechnology industry and Big Pharma as central players in medicalization, signal a new urgency in interrogating medicalization and its mental health counterpart, psychiatrization. These shifts direct attention to the systemic antecedents of the medicalization process and its perpetuation of oppressive structures and economic processes that create and sustain mental health struggles in oppressed peoples.

Intergenerational Trauma Transmission and Oppressed Peoples

The chapter would not be complete without an emphasis on the central importance of intergenerational trauma transmission in oppressed peoples. As the evidence throughout this book attests, oppression inscribes deep physical, spiritual and psychological wounds caused by processes such as the misogyny inherent in violence against women and girls, the legacy of slavery in the United States and Canada and the imperialism that has led to Canada's economic apartheid against racialized peoples. Trauma is, by its nature, deeply embedded in the soul, the psyche and the cognitive schema of those who are traumatized. The world may become reframed as a dangerous place, and continued survival often involves feelings of detachment or numbing. Recurring images and nightmares of traumatic experiences create a persistent reliving of the trauma(s)(Herman, 1997). The impact of oppression-related trauma on individuals and families has been described extensively in the feminist therapy literature, the first field to link psychological trauma with oppressive societal structures.

There is remarkably little literature about the ways that oppression-based trauma is threaded through generations of oppressed peoples. Although it is well recognized that parental experiences can have a lasting impact on children, public policymakers, practitioners and researchers in the health fields have barely begun to understand or acknowledge the notion that the traumatization of a whole people can be transmitted through generations. According to Kira (2001), intergenerational trauma transmission includes the following three areas: generational family trauma transmission; collective, cross-generational trauma transmission; and multigenerational transmission of structural violence. In generational family trauma transmission, adults' traumatic experiences and their effects get transmitted within a family system across generations. In Canada, Indian residential school survivors were persistently under threat of, and endured, incarceration, starvation, physical and sexual abuse, and even torture. This brutal treatment severely impacted their adult lives and their parenting over time (Paul, 2006), thus creating the context for family trauma transmission. There is no doubt that the way that Aboriginal people remember their past and interpret those events, as individuals and as a people, contributes to contemporary social problems in Aboriginal communities (Wesley-Esquimaux & Smolewski, 2004).

These Indigenous family struggles related to Indian residential schools happened in synergy with collective, cross-generational trauma transmission. According to Kira (2001), trauma is best described as a collective complex trauma when it is inflicted on a group of people with specific group identity or affiliation to ethnicity, colour, national origin or religion. Kira points out that this kind of trauma tends to be ignored in most clinical assessment and treatment. When a whole group of people is traumatized persistently over decades and indeed centuries, the impact of this trauma carries on through generations, like a thread or a web of threads. In the dedication of Dr. Daniel Paul's (2006: 5) book, *We Were Not the Savages*, he eloquently refers to this traumatization and the strong survival of the Mi'Kmaq people:

> To the memory of my ancestors, who managed to ensure the survival of the Mi'Kmaq people by their awe-inspiring tenacity and valour in the face of virtually insurmountable odds! For more than four centuries these courageous, dignified and heroic people displayed a determination to survive the various hells on earth created for them by Europeans with a tenacity that equals any displayed in the history of mankind. May their brave accomplishment inspire the Mi'Kmaq and other oppressed peoples to meet the challenges of today and tomorrow.

The groundbreaking work of Cynthia Wesley-Esquimaux and Maglalena Smolewski (2004), built on psychological trauma theory and the writings of Judith Herman (1992), presents a critical analysis of the psychological transmission of oppression-based trauma in Aboriginal peoples (McGibbon & Etowa, 2009). These authors described the near extinction of many Aboriginal peoples through contact with disease-carrying Europeans during the early period of colonization. For societies in North America, first contact probably occurred around 1500. Therefore, Aboriginal peoples in Canada have survived over five centuries of colonization. These centuries of cultural dispossession, cultural genocide, including loss of Indigenous languages, and physical brutality are embedded in the Aboriginal psyche. Social and health problems of Aboriginal people have roots in extensive historical trauma that society has never properly acknowledged (Wesley-Esquimaux, Smolewski 2009: 53):

> The meta-narrative of the Western world simply did not include the entire Aboriginal story of loss and impermanence. Collectively, one may refer to Aboriginal people as the "bereaved": those who have been deprived of something dear — their cultural identity and their social self. Bereavement is always associated with grief. If one

perceives loss as separating oneself from a part of life to which one was emotionally attached, Aboriginal grief may be understood as an attempt to restore equilibrium to their social system. It involves all of the emotional, cognitive and perceptual reactions that accompany such loss. Ideally it should be followed by a recovery that involves survivors restructuring their lives.

The centrality of cultural, spiritual and material loss is a cornerstone of intergenerational trauma transmission among oppressed peoples. The most well-developed research and writings about intergenerational trauma transmission include the psychotherapeutic work with Nazi Holocaust survivors. Another important area of knowledge includes the truth and reconciliation process in post-apartheid South Africa. The slavery of American and Canadian Black people and the Armenian genocide in Turkey are also examples of horrific experiences that have created intergenerational or historical trauma transmission. Gump (2010: Abstract) discusses intergenerational trauma transmission in African-Americans, noting that few psychoanalytic theories accord social, political and cultural realities a role in the development of the psyche:

> This silence distorts and constricts our understanding of all subjects, but is particularly pernicious for the nondominant, as it renders significant aspects of their subjectivities invisible. African American subjectivity is an instance of such omission. The trauma of slavery critically shaped our subjectivity, yet this impact is rarely acknowledged. In fact, the subjugation, cruelties, and deprivations of slavery have given a traumatic cast to African American subjectivity. Through the intergenerational transmission of trauma this wounding has endured. (Gump, 2010)

Multigenerational transmission of structural violence creates extreme social disparities (Kira, 2001). These systemic structures and their impacts on oppressed people are described in detail in Chapter 12. Poverty, biologically induced traumas such as hunger or prolonged malnutrition, inadequate and crowded shelter, inadequate medical care, unemployment, underemployment or employment in temporary jobs without fringe benefits all cause severe mental health consequences over time. They can cause parental insecurity; overwork; fatigue and accompanying irritability; limited availability of parents to children because of overwork; fatigue, tension and illness; and chronic ongoing threats to security and well-being for parents and children (Kira, 2001). As might be expected, the three forms of intergenerational trauma described here (generational family trauma transmission; collective, cross-generational trauma transmission; and multigenerational transmission of structural violence) can and do happen together. Indeed, as the discussion in this chapter attests, cross-generational trauma is linked in a complex way to the structural, oppression-based antecedents of ill health.

Judith Herman's (1992: xvi) formulation of complex trauma greatly illuminates our understanding of intergenerational trauma: "The beauty of the complex post traumatic stress disorder concept is in its integrative nature. Rather than a simple list of symptoms, it is a coherent formulation of the consequences of prolonged and repeated trauma." Herman's description of the two main underpinnings of complex trauma helps us to understand the political and relational meanings of intergenerational trauma. First, complex trauma is "always embedded in a social structure that permits the abuse and exploitation of a subordinate group" (xiv). As many of the chapters in this book argue, systemic social structures embedded in political ideologies, and consequently in public policy, create and sustain repeated traumas for oppressed people over time. Second, complex trauma "is always relational. It takes place when the victim is in a state of captivity, under the control and domination of the perpetrator" (xiv). Herman's description of the victim-perpetrator relationship is analogous to the five-century-long European occupation of the Americas and the centuries-old capture, displacement and intergenerational brutality perpetrated by European slave traders on peoples of the African diaspora.

Conclusions

The layers and structures involved in moving the anti-oppressive project forward in the area of mental health are far-reaching and complex. This is because the everyday implementation of psychiatrization, by actual people in actual geographies (human relationships), is articulated to the larger structural relations of biomedical and biotechnological systems and capitalism and market-driven health care (social or ruling relations), as described in Chapter 1. The way forward necessarily happens in both of these realms.

A robust critique of biomedical dominance and psychiatry have been evident in the literature for many decades, so much so that critiques of psychiatry became known as "anti-psychiatry." However, while critical social scientists have been advancing the critique of psychiatry and its modern-day capitalist iterations, the field itself and the ways it operates in clinical and institutional settings have become even more entrenched in psychiatrization. These two worlds (critical social science and psychiatry) are largely parallel and must be integrated if we are to move forward in addressing SDH inequities that are at the root of many, if not most, mental health struggles. More accurately, psychiatric approaches must be interrogated and, wherever necessary, amended or discarded to bring a subjective and historically informed compassion to practice, education and public policy.

10

Oppression, Health and Public Policy in Canada

Toba Bryant

Public policy may be defined as action or inaction by governments to address what has been identified as a public issue (Wolf, 2005). Public policy is anchored in a set of values about appropriate public goals and a set of beliefs about how to achieve those goals (Pal, 2006). Health policy is a subset of public policy that is intended to address a range of health-related issues such as resource allocation for the delivery of health care. Health policy is also concerned with improving and maintaining the health of a population and therefore the distribution of social and economic resources such as income, housing, education and employment, among others, to the population (CPHI, 2004b).

Public policy is usually thought of as the means by which governments strive to meet the needs of the population. Increasingly, however, it would seem that public policy frequently creates barriers that prevent vulnerable populations from accessing social determinants of health such as income, housing and food. As a result, these populations experience insecurity, which has implications for their health and well-being. In these cases, public policy can be seen as creating practices and conditions of oppression.

Oppression has been defined as both a state and a process (Prilletensky & Gonick, 1996). As a state or outcome, oppressive conditions occur when access to resources has been consistently denied (Watts & Abdul-Adil, 1994). The condition of oppression usually refers to a state of domination in which those who are oppressed endure deprivation, exclusion, discrimination and exploitation (Bartky, 1990; Prilletensky & Gonick, 1996; Sidanius, 1993). As a process, oppression usually entails institutionalized collective and individual forms of behaviour by which one group exerts domination and control over another (Mar'i, 1988). The intent is usually to derive some political, economic or other advantage over another group.

For the purposes of this chapter, oppression is both a condition and a process created by public policies that systematically deny some members of society access to economic and social resources. This chapter argues that public policy can oppress by creating practices and conditions that deny some populations access to the social determinants of health, such as housing, employment and food security, among others. It is possible to identify different levels of oppression by comparing the extent and quality of social and health provision to citizens in several countries. based on the levels of social and health provision to citizens.

Oppression and Public Policy

A substantial literature examines the political and psychological dimensions of oppression, recognizing that it is not possible to consider one in isolation from the other (Bartky, 1990). As indicated, oppression is a state and also involves practices and conditions in which access to the social determinants of health is consistently withheld by one group from another in society (Mar'i, 1988; Watts & Abdul-Adil, 1994). Prilletensky and Gonick (1996) argue that oppression can be understood at several levels of analysis, including micro and macro. Micro analysis is concerned with individual perceptions of self worth as inadequate or inferior to others and feelings of powerlessness. Macro analyses direct attention to political and economic structures at national and global levels, or public policies that impinge on people's lives. These authors argue that a more complete analysis of oppression would link political and psychological analyses, thereby recognizing how these levels interact. Both the political and psychological "domains" must be recognized in order to "reduce conditions of oppression" (128). Perhaps less well understood are the connections between oppression and public policy. Specifically, how does public policy create practices and conditions of oppression? If we are to understand the impact of public policy, we must consider what public policy is intended to do and for whose benefit.

What Is Public Policy?

As aforementioned, public policy is a course of action undertaken by government to address a social problem or interrelated set of problems (Pal, 2006). Health policy is a subset of public policy that is concerned with the allocation and management of resources within the health care system. It is also concerned with improving and maintaining the health of a population by ensuring access to social and economic resources for health and social well-being. The form public policy takes is strongly influenced by a range of factors. Theories of public policy development can explicate the various dimensions of the public policy process. These theories are usually classified in one of two potential categories: consensus and conflict (Brooks & Miljan, 2003a; Walt, 1994).

Consensus Theories

Consensus theoretical approaches tend to focus on how various groups vie with one another to influence the public policymaking process and realize their policy objectives. Such theories assume that public policy is developed on the basis of a rational consideration of all of the potential options for addressing a given public issue. Government then usually decides on the course of action based on a cost and benefit analysis. Many applied models of public policy were developed on assumptions drawn from the physical and natural sciences. Early public policy theorists applied these models with the intent to improve the quality of public policy decisions and to make the public policy realm more like science (Albaek, 1995; Brunner, 1991).

Pluralism, an example of a consensus theory and one of the most influential theories of public policy in North America, refers to the numerous ways of thinking about policy issues that exist in any given society (Signal, 1998; Walt, 1994). Pluralism conceives politics as involving a "plurality" of interest groups competing with one another to influence public policy outcomes (Walt, 1994). It assumes a level playing field for all groups attempting to influence the public policymaking process. No one elite is considered to dominate the political process at any time. Pluralist concepts emphasize evidence and ideas and how professional and citizen groups build support for a particular approach to public policymaking. This analysis assumes,that advocates wanting to reduce social and health inequalities will not face undue resistance from governments to their ideas concerning inequality and oppression, and that influencing policymakers to address the root causes of decreased access to the sdh, for example, will not present special problems.

Conflict or Materialist Theories

Conflict approaches direct attention to political ideology, values and power in shaping how governments and societies respond to social problems — if at all — and how those problems are defined (Brooks & Miljan, 2003b). In other words, conflict theories are concerned with how political and economic forces, such as political ideology and powerful economic interests, influence public policy. They are also concerned specifically with the distribution of power within a society. Thus, public policymaking often does not reflect the validity of evidence and ideas but rather the undue influence of powerful economic and political interests. The dominant political ideology — a set of ideas about how to address a public problem or set of interrelated problems –defines how government responds to issues. For example, concepts such as the social determinants of health will be resisted since they may adversely affect those who profit from low wages, lack of affordable housing and the private provision of child care. These theories are therefore more appropriate for understanding how conditions and practices of oppression develop.

Materialism is an example of a conflict, or critical, theory of public policy. It focuses on political, economic and social structures — such as the political

ideology of society and the distribution of economic and social resources —
and considers that society is based on conflict, not consensus (Bourgeault,
2006). In other words, materialism and political economy provide macro or
structural analyses of issues. Politics and economics are seen as interrelated
and as shaping the organization and distribution of social and economic
resources such as income, housing, education and health care in a society
(Armstrong & Armstrong, 2003; Coburn, 2006). Attributes such as gender,
social class, race and sexual orientation are considered to negatively affect
access to the social determinants of health and to political power. Unequal
distribution of resources results in unequal health outcomes for different
groups based on social class, gender, race and other attributes.

Materialism, or a materialist political economy, considers the role of
political ideology, public policies, practices and conditions of a society in
oppressing certain groups (Armstrong, 2006). Political ideology is seen as
fundamentally shaping public policies that lead to particular practices and
conditions, thereby influencing social and health outcomes. For example, if
the political party in power believes that it has a role to play in ensuring that
all citizens have access to a decent income, housing and education, and related
programs and services, then it will enact policies and invest financial resources
to to ensure that these resources are available as a right of citizenship. Such
redistributive ideas are more consistent with social democratic — rather than
liberal — ideology that is committed to redistributive policies, or policies that
ensure all citizens have access to resources such as education and health care,
regardless of their income. Critical theories are therefore more appropriate
for understanding political and social outcomes in society. In particular, they
enable consideration of the form of the welfare state in a country and the
level of provision by government to a population.

During the past two decades, Canada's capacity to address health
inequalities by way of their underlying social determinants has weakened
(Grieshaber-Otto & Sinclair, 2004; Teeple, 2000). While health spending has
remained relatively constant, social spending has substantially decreased.
There are two stylized explanations of how these policy directions came
about: (1) inadequate or ineffective knowledge generation, dissemination and translation; and (2) changes in Canada's political and economic
economy, partly related to increased integration into the world economy
and associated with shifting political allegiances and values. The first explanation is consistent with a consensus or pluralist perspective. The second
explanation is consistent with a conflict perspective. Recent public policy
changes have increased social inequalities and reduced access to social and
economic resources. The following sections examine the changes that have
occurred through the lens of the welfare state as a vehicle for reducing the
likelihood of oppression.

Growth in Social and Health Inequalities in Canada

Since the 1970s, social and economic changes have altered the global economy (Grieshaber-Otto & Sinclair, 2004; Teeple, 2000). Governments in Canada, the United Kingdom, the United States and elsewhere have reduced the share of national wealth allocated to social and health spending, justifying these reductions as ensuring their global economic competitiveness. This process has occurred in tandem with the deregulation of markets and reduced government interventions in the working of the economy. These changes have contributed to growing income inequality in developed and developing economies (OECD, 2008). In fact, Canada has had one of the largest increases in inequality among developed political economies.

Much research shows that the effects of deregulated markets and reduced government interventions in the workings of the marketplace may not be beneficial or even benign, as reflected in growing social and health inequalities (Leys, 2001; Macarov, 2003; McBride & Shields, 1997). Some countries have resisted the demands of globalization by maintaining consistent and high public spending on health and social programs. Other economies, however, seem to be more susceptible — indeed receptive — to market domination and have lowered the proportion of national wealth devoted to social and health care provision to citizens (OECD, 2008, 2007a).

Comparison of spending on health and social programs can illustrate key differences in the extent of the welfare state and its capacity to reduce social and health inequalities. Such analysis shows that those nations identified as market-dominated political economies tend to transfer fewer national resources toward social and health provision to the citizenry. In these countries, citizens are much more dependent upon paid labour to ensure their well-being. The result is that wages and benefits lag behind the situation in nations where governmental transfers are more generous (Raphael, 2007b). The combination of market deregulation and reduced government intervention and spending creates conditions of oppression. In other words, the welfare state — government intervention into the social and health policy fields — helps to ensure access to key social and economic resources that are necessary to maintain the health and well-being of populations, particularly for low-income and other vulnerable households.

Theoretical Frameworks of the Welfare State

Several theoretical frameworks have been devised to understand how public policy components fit together to define a specific type of welfare state. Esping-Andersen's typology of capitalist welfare states — social democratic, conservative and liberal — has generated much attention and research (Esping-Andersen, 1990, 2002). The social democratic welfare states have high social and health spending and provide more generous support to citizens. Such regimes have as an objective to reduce inequalities and poverty in a population (Saint-Arnaud & Bernard, 2003). Exemplars of the social democratic welfare state are Sweden, Norway, Denmark and usually Finland (Bambra, 2007).

In contrast, liberal welfare states tend to have lower public spending on health and social programs. Canada, the United States, the United Kingdom, Australia and New Zealand are exemplars of this type of regime. Canada's welfare-oriented policies show strong similarities to the other nations in the liberal cluster. While Canada differs from the United States in many of its public policies, in a broader perspective that includes other wealthy developed nations, it is closer to the United States in its welfare provision than to social democratic nations, or to conservative nations such as France and Germany. Canada is similar to social democratic regimes only in its public health care provision — and even then the public system covers fewer health care needs than is the case in social democratic nations (OECD, 2007a). Conservative welfare states tend to fall between the social democratic and liberal welfare states in their public spending on social and health programs (Bambra, 2009).

Esping-Andersen's typology is useful for illustrating the differences among nations, particularly with respect to their capacity to reduce the gap between high- and low-income groups and reduce poverty in the new global economy. Figure 10.1 illustrates a scheme devised by Saint-Arnaud and Bernard (2003) to identify the key institutions and dominant values and political ideology that define each type of welfare state. Their analysis provides many insights into the operation of these political economies and how they shape public policy.

As we can see, the dominant institution in liberal welfare states is the market, and the dominant value is liberty, or freedom from government (Ham & Hill, 1984; Saint-Arnaud & Bernard, 2003). Its main organizing principle is residual, that is, focused on providing for the immediate needs of the most disadvantaged. In contrast, the dominant institution in social democratic welfare states is the state, the dominant value is equality, and the primary organizing principle is universalism. In conservative regimes, solidarity is the key ideology. Its main organizing principle is insurance for access to benefits, which are dependent on previous contributions made by employer and employee to benefits programs. The dominant institution in a conservative regime is the family. These conceptualizations are consistent with Esping-Andersen's original assertion that social democratic regimes have a central objective of reducing social and health inequalities — including poverty and disadvantage — among income groups. The relationships among these typologies and pubic policy are further explored in Chapter 12.

Figure 10.1: Ideological Variations in Forms of the Welfare State

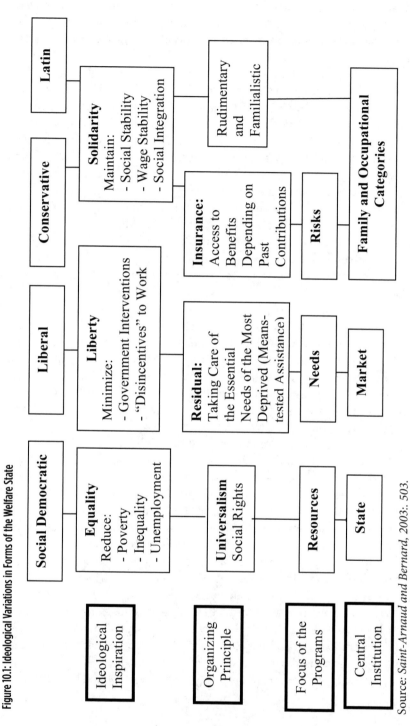

Source: Saint-Arnaud and Bernard, 2003:. 503.

Social Inequalities and the Welfare State

Social inequality refers to the unequal distribution of social and economic resources in a society (Grabb, 2007). The degree or depth of inequality in a society is directly related to government spending on social and health programs such as health care, income support during periods of unemployment, social assistance and other income support programs. It is also related to financial investment in education and employment training, the latter usually termed "active labour policy" (OECD, 2007b). Government spending ensures that all citizens have equal access to social and economic resources such as income, housing, education and employment. In the political economy literature, the term given to making these resources available as a matter of right — rather than subject to purchase on the market — is "decommodification" (Coburn, 2006; Esping-Andersen, 1990). To deny access to these resources constitutes a form of oppression, resulting in economic and social marginalization of some populations, particularly those who have low incomes.

Public policies that promote the redistribution of income and other resources from high-income to low-income groups help to reduce social and health inequalities in a society (Teeple, 2000). The most obvious evidence of this is the extent of poverty present within a nation (Brady, 2003). The package of public policies that serve to redistribute income and reduce social and health inequalities within populations has come to be known as the welfare state. In nations such as Canada, the United States and the United Kingdom, the post-World War II welfare state enabled the intervention by government in the workings of the economic system to provide programs such as health care, social assistance and housing as rights of citizenship (Esping-Andersen, 2002; Teeple, 2000). The creation of the welfare state signified a victory for the working class in exacting from government provisions that would provide security to individuals and families during periods of unemployment (Teeple, 2000). Comparing government spending in Canada with spending in other countries illustrates growing inequality in Canada and hence increased oppression of low-income populations. The following discussion shows that Canada has among the lowest social and health spending levels among the developed economies.

Governments make decisions on what proportion of a country's gross domestic product (GDP) to allocate to a broad range of health and social programs. These programs include cash payments, benefits in-kind and allocations of spending on pensions, disability, active labour market policies, families and health care. The OECD regularly publishes indicators of these government expenditures. A particularly important indicator is that of government transfers, which refers to governments using fiscal resources generated by the economy and distributing them to the population in the form of services, income supports or investments in social infrastructure. Such infrastructure can include education, employment training, social assistance, family supports, pensions, health and social services, and specific benefits such as free or subsidized housing or government-funded or subsidized drug coverage. The following sections examine government social spending and spending on cash and in-kind benefits.

Social Spending

Figure 10.2 shows overall social spending as a percentage of GDP for nations that are members of the Organization for Economic Cooperation and Development for 2003, the most recent year for which data is available (OECD, 2008). Among OECD member countries, the total net social expenditure was just over 23 percent of GDP in 2003. France, a conservative political economy, spends 31 percent of its GDP on social programs. Sweden, a social democratic political economy, spends just over 29 percent. Canada and the US rank near the bottom in social spending. Both countries hovered below 20 percent in both 2001 and 2003, just ahead of Ireland, Mexico and Korea who have very low spending levels of around 10 percent of GDP.

Figure 10.2 Total Public Expenditure as % of GDP, 2003

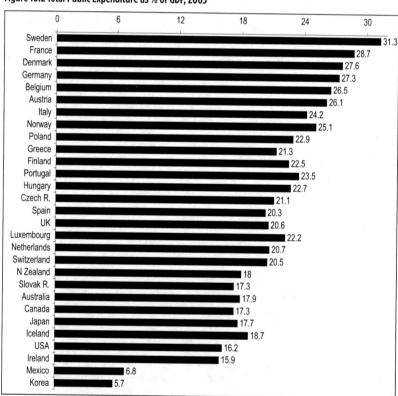

Source: *From Social Expenditure Database, 2008, Paris:* OECD.

Income Transfers and Benefits In-Kind

Cash and benefits in-kind are social benefits that in market-oriented nations serve to reduce social inequality. Cash refers to income such as social assistance, unemployment insurance and other income paid out in government transfers to citizens as a matter of right (e.g., universal child benefits) or directed to those in need (e.g., social assistance or welfare). Benefits in-kind refer to non-cash reimbursements, such as prescription medications, child-care subsidies or free or subsidized housing. Among OECD member nations, Sweden and France spend nearly 20 percent of their GDP on income transfers and just under 15 percent on benefits-in-kind. Canada and the United States fall well behind these leaders. Canada spends less than 8 percent on cash benefits and less than 10 percent of its GDP on in-kind benefits (see Figure 10.3).

The U.S. spends around 8 percent on cash benefits and less than 8 percent on benefits in-kind. In contrast, the social democratic states, known for their

Figure 10.3 Cash and Benefits-in-Kind as % of GDP, 2003

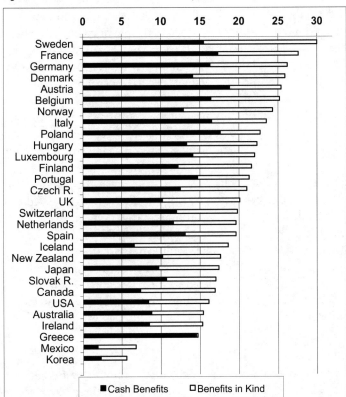

Source: *From Social Expenditure Database*, OECD *2008, Paris:* OECD.

cradle-to-grave welfare state, exceed the spending of most other nations, while both Canada and the United States are among the lowest spenders. Social democratic welfare regimes have relatively less conditions of oppression since goods and services are highly decommodified. In other words, the state provides necessary goods and services, instead of citizens having to rely on their market incomes to purchase them.

Implications of Reduced Government Spending

The extent of the welfare state — or social and health provision –in countriescan provide insights into the types of policies and practices of governments. The degree to which these services are decommodified indicates the extent of oppression for vulnerable households and populations in a country. Canada's low spending has led to high levels of inequality. Although Canada has decommodified health care and some social services, it has marketized some health services, which has implications for access to these services.

Inequality is a form of oppression. In this sense oppression can be equated with a process of social and economic marginalization. Considerable research shows that the groups most likely to experience social and economic marginalization are racialized, that is, they are people of colour (Galabuzi, 2001; Ornstein, 2000). These groups lack access to basic social and economic goods such as a living wage, housing and employment security, among others. Galabuzi refers to this condition as social exclusion: groups of people are deprived access to basic social and economic resources, thereby depriving them of the opportunity to be fully participating citizens in ways that are normally expected in modern democracies. Chapter 7 further explores the nature of social exclusion and its enduring impact on health and well-being.

In recent years, much has been written about the impact of less government regulation of the market on social and health inequalities. The emergence of neoliberalism as the dominant political ideology has led to a reduced government role in housing and other social policy areas. Indeed, critics consider that public policies shaped by neoliberal principles lead to oppressive practices and conditions that result in deteriorating social conditions, or growing social and health inequalities. Changes in Canada's political and economic economy — partly related to increased integration into the world economy and associated with shifting political allegiances and values — have contributed to this situation.

Conclusion

Oppression is the denial of access to social and economic resources in a society. Public policies — in particular spending by governments on social and health programs — can lead to oppressive practices and conditions. Oppression is social exclusion of vulnerable populations. The growth of income inequality since the 1970s has been particularly pronounced in Canada, the United States, the United Kingdom and other countries defined as liberal welfare states. Liberal welfare states seem to be particularly likely to reduce government spending and commodify goods and services, leading to high levels of inequality and oppressive conditions for vulnerable populations. In contrast, social democratic welfare regimes provide more generous supports to citizens and are less likely to create oppressive practices and conditions. Liberal welfare regimes appear to be particularly susceptible to the impact of economic globalization — and hence neoliberalism — as they seem willing to deregulate and reduce health and social spending to enhance their competitiveness in the new global economy.

The result is a growing concentration of wealth, increasing inequalities and increased oppression for low-income and other vulnerable populations. The solution to oppression is to implement public policies more consistent with social democratic principles of equity and social justice. This will require the building of social and political movements that will force policymakers to develop and implement public policies consistent with such principles.

A Rights-Based Approach to Primary Health Care

Increasing Accountability for Health Inequities within Health Systems Strengthening

Charmaine McPherson

It is my aspiration that health finally will be seen not as a blessing to be wished for, but as a human right to be fought for. — *Kofi Annan, former United Nations Secretary-General*

No analysis of oppression and health would be complete without considering the possibilities that exist within health systems strengthening through a primary health care framework. There is growing interest in united action in achieving "health for all" through primary health care, with its focus on health as a human right and social justice. Recent global discourse has focused on "health systems strengthening" as a national policy strategy. This simply means that health systems need to be reformed to be strong enough to be able to provide citizens with the health services needed to deliver on equitable health outcomes. In this chapter, health systems strengthening is connected with primary health care renewal as a comprehensive approach to public system strengthening. Ideally, health outcomes, interventions, programs and systems come together in a robust national health policy and strategy (WHO, 2010a). However, it is generally recognized that neither the state nor the private sector are sufficiently accountable to support effective and equitable service provision (Gauri, 2003). Preferably, accountability structures and processes would help to determine what is working, so that it can be repeated, and what is not, so that it can be adjusted (Hunt, 2007). Health systems strengthening through primary health care renewal needs clearer and effective accountability that is connected to broadly understood and accepted principles and processes, which, in turn, are consistent with primary health care ideals. A human rights-based approach may provide such a framework.

"Health for all" is a laudable goal. So, why do governments and their agents knowingly continue to foster oppression within health care and other public service systems? Why are wealthy nations struggling with the realization of primary health care? How can and should nations move towards the ideals of health for all? Although this chapter may pose more questions than it answers, the primary focus is on uncovering and addressing health-impacting oppression within an agenda focused on health systems strengthening through primary health care. Core concepts are considered and the linkages among health, health equity and a human rights-based approach to health service planning and policy development are examined. The discussion then outlines how a rights-based approach may be embedded in reformative primary health care policy and programming and also analyzes key major issues hindering this transformation. The chapter closes with some promising directions for a way forward on the issues of health inequities and primary health care renewal.

Health Equity, Primary Health Care and a Human Rights-Based Approach

Within human rights discourse, the principle of "equity" increasingly serves as an important nonlegal generic policy term aimed at ensuring fairness. The term has been used to embrace policy-related issues such as service access and affordability (Nygren-Krug, 2008). The focused attention on vulnerable and disadvantaged groups in society in international human rights instruments reinforces the principle of equity. "Health equity" means the absence of systematic disparities in health, or in the major social determinants of health, between groups with different levels of underlying social advantage or disadvantage — that is, wealth, power or prestige (Braveman & Gruskin, 2003). Health equity is a basic principle of primary health care.

Primary health care is about providing essential health care that is based on the needs of the population, that is universally accessible to individuals and families in the community and that is provided as close as possible to where people live and work. Primary health care is decentralized and requires the active participation of the community and family (WHO, 1978). Primary health care has been around for more than fifty years. The concept became popularized after the WHO enshrined it in the 1978 Declaration of Alma-Ata. Fundamental to the primary health care philosophy of health for all are a social value system and principles that include notions of people-centredness, equity, efficiency, sustainability, community engagement, social justice, prevention, solidarity, cross-sectoral early intervention and economic and social productivity. These principles translate into equitable, comprehensive and universal basic health care; protection of the most vulnerable in our society; the use of empowering and participatory processes in health service and policy development and implementation; and health improvement efforts that must address and integrate the social determinants of health (WHO, 1978). The Declaration of Alma-Ata marked the start of a new paradigm for improving public health and provided a new platform for international health policy (Periago, 2007). The principles of the declaration were built on a fundamental premise of primary health care: health is a basic human right.

We talk about primary health care *renewal* because there has been as renewed emphasis on achieving effective primary health care globally, as outlined in the 1978 declaration, especially since the release of the *World Health Report* in 2008 (WHO, 2008b). It is generally accepted that primary health care must be an integral part of health systems development and reform and that basing health systems on primary health care is the best approach for producing sustained and equitable improvement in citizens' health. A primary health care-based health system is an overarching approach to the organization and operation of health systems that makes the right to the highest attainable level of health its main goal while maximizing equity and solidarity (Macinko, Montenagro, & Nebot, 2007; McPherson & McGibbon, 2010a).

Essential to the Alma-Ata's primary health care approach was the denunciation of the gross inequities in the health status of the people both between and within countries. At the time, this situation was seen as politically, socially and economically unacceptable (WHO, 1978). These inequities and the call for change is as real today as it was in 1978, in all countries — northern and southern; low, middle and high income countries alike. "It would be wrong to suggest that a primary health care approach would 'solve' all problems of services delivery, but at least the orientation of the services would have some chance of addressing population need in humane and effective ways… challenging the dominant paradigm of [western] medicine and health care delivery" (Macdonald, 2004, p. 285). The primary health care vision contains an implicit critique of western health systems — with a downstream, medico-technical orientation and division between treatment and prevention/health promotion (Macdonald, 2004).

A human rights based approach (RBA) has been recognized as a major way to advance equality in many fields; it provides a discourse with a visionary framework as well as a useful guide for analysis and action. Human rights provide accepted international norms and standards, such as definitions of concepts and attention to particular vulnerable population groups. An RBA moves decision-makers beyond averages to focus on those groups in society that are considered most vulnerable (e.g., Indigenous peoples, women and children living in poverty); it provides the deliberate opportunity to advance specific human rights to protect these vulnerable populations. Examples include the right to full information and the right to participate in decisions affecting their own health. Human rights thus form a strong basis for policymakers and health systems to prioritize the health needs of vulnerable and marginalized populations — priority groups within primary health care.

Many variations on a human rights-based approach are evolving and there are also critiques of these various methods. Developing innovative and effective ways to apply RBA principles is a work in progress, especially in the health field. There are, however, fundamental principles embedded in an RBA, as outlined in the Stamford Common Understanding (UNESCO, 2003). Box 11.1 provides a useful acronym, PANEL, for talking about RBA principles.

The PANEL analysis is a simplified version of a more comprehensive approach that is outlined in internationally accepted sources (e.g., UNIFEM, the United Nations Development Fund for Women). Notably, the UNESCO, in its strategy on human rights for the social and human sciences, recommended that, of the five principles, non-discrimination is the one that should lead to operational change (Frankovits, 2006).

Box 11.1 PANEL: Human Rights Based Approach Principles

Participation — Recognizes people as key actors in their own development rather than passive recipients of commodities and services; participation is both a means and a goal; analysis includes all stakeholders; strategic partnerships are developed and sustained.

Accountability — Requires development of laws and administrative procedures, practices and mechanisms to ensure fulfillment of entitlements, as well as opportunities to address denials and violations; calls for translation of universal standards into locally determined benchmarks for measuring progress and enhancing accountability.

Non-discrimination and Equality — Requires particular focus on addressing discrimination and inequality, focusing on marginalized, disadvantaged and excluded groups.

Empowerment — Process by which people's capabilities to demand and use their human rights grows; they are empowered to claim their rights rather than simply wait for policies, legislation or provision of services; development process is locally owned.

Linkages to Human Rights Standards — Programming informed by recommendations of international human rights bodies and mechanisms.

Source: Adapted from Tomas (2005)

Linkages among Health,
Health Equity and Human Rights

The right to the highest attainable standard of health, referred to as the "right to health," was first reflected in 1946 in the WHO Constitution and was reiterated in the 1978 Declaration of Alma-Ata (WHO, 1978) and again in the World Health Declaration adopted by the World Health Assembly in 1998 (Nygren-Krug, 2008). Although the Alma-Ata (WHO, 1978) drew the connection between primary health care and health as a human right, the right to health does not mean the right to be healthy, nor does it mean that poor governments must offer expensive health services that they cannot resource. The right to health *does* require governments and public authorities to develop and administer policies and action plans that will lead to available and accessible health care for all in the shortest possible time. This is a challenge given the relative disconnect between the human rights and health worlds: "Health and wellbeing have not always been at the forefront of human rights discussions and, conversely, public health agencies too infrequently consider the human rights dimensions of their work" (Periago, 2007, p. 1).

Health is essential to wellbeing and to overcoming other effects of social disadvantage. If there was health equity, then people's needs, rather than their social privileges, would guide the distribution of opportunities for well-being. This means eliminating disparities in health and in health's major determinants that are systematically associated with underlying social disadvantage within a society (Raphael, 2009a).

The distinct and complex linkages and synergies among health, health equity and human rights (McPherson & McGibbon, 2010a; McGibbon & Etowa, 2009) constitute the fundamental idea of the health and human rights movement. Human rights and public health have the common objectives of promoting and protecting the well-being of all individuals. Human rights must be promoted and protected in order to address the underlying determinants of health (WHO, 2007c, p. 1). Inequities in health systematically breach basic human rights and put groups of people who are already socially marginalized and oppressed at further disadvantage regarding their health.

Jonathan Mann, a central advocate of combining the synergistic forces of public health, ethics and human rights, drew the connection between health and human rights as two distinct yet inseparable realities (Mann, et al., 1999). Mann and colleagues argue that access to quality health care is a self-evident, inalienable right shared by all human beings, as recognized by the United Nations Universal Declaration of Human Rights. There is an "inextricable connection" between health and human rights such that "promoting and protecting health requires explicit and concrete efforts to promote and to protect human rights and dignity, and greater fulfillment of human rights necessitates sound attention to health and its societal determinants" (Mann et al., 1999, p. 5).

Human rights violations are underlying causes of adverse health outcomes for vulnerable people and populations around the world (Beyrer & Pizer, 2007). Some experts even claim that our very humanity is threatened by our collective failure to end such abuses, including insidious human rights violations caused by structural violence involving the denial of basic requirements for health, such as economic opportunities, decent housing, education and access to health care (Farmer, 2003). This situation is not the result of random events — it is the result of bad public policy decisions on many levels or good decisions that were badly implemented across many public sectors (Lipsky, 1980; Pressman & Wildavsky, 1984). If we accept that public policies may be defined as anything a government chooses to do or not do (Dye, 1972), then, put simply, choices made by public decision-makers are at the root of developing and maintaining health inequities. Primary health care offers an opportunity for public system decision-makers to alleviate the very oppression brought on by ineffective or absent policy or by poor policy implementation — through a countering policy and service implementation philosophy that is based on social justice.

Equitable health outcomes are the ultimate measure of a well-performing health system. Primary health care was designed to achieve equitable and sustainable health development. In reality, one might say that primary health care was an attempt to fight some of the oppressive forces brought on by the very public services that should have protected people. However, particular populations continue to experience clear health inequities that are often associated with human rights abuses, and the Alma-Ata vision is disappointingly far from reach.

A Rights-Based Approach to Furthering Health Equity

The right to health and the conditions necessary for health have been firmly endorsed in a wide range of international and regional human rights instruments, such as the International Convention on the Rights of the Child (United Nations, 1989) and the Convention on the Elimination of All Forms of Discrimination Against Women (United Nations, 1979). Every WHO member state has ratified (formally consented to be legally bound by) at least one human rights treaty, all of which have direct or indirect bearing on the promotion and protection of the right to health and health-related rights, including the right to conditions necessary for health (WHO, 2007c; 2010c). The most authoritative recent interpretation of the right to health is outlined in Article 12 of the International Covenant on Economic, Social and Cultural

Table 11.1 Declarations and Resolutions Made by Ministers of Health of the Americas Recognizing Links among Health, Human Rights and Health Systems Strengthening

Instrument	Date	Significance of Instrument
Declaration of Caracas	November 14, 1990	PAHO's initial work on human rights in collaboration with regional human rights bodies; First inter-American standard to directly link international human rights conventions to psychiatric patient rights; recommended legislative renewal to ensure rights protection.
Vienna Declaration *and Programme of Action*	June 1993	Adopted at Vienna World Conference on Human Rights; declared that all U.N. bodies and specialized agencies are required to periodically assess impact of their policies and strategies on enjoyment of human rights.
Resolution on Disability	September 25, 1999	Approved by 35 PAHO member states; officially recognized human rights conventions and standards as essential tools for restructuring health systems; called for collaboration among national, regional and international human rights bodies.
Declaration of Mar Del Plata	June 17, 2005	Developed at meeting of Ministers of Health and Environment of the Americas (HEMA); recognized need for civil society organizations among major groups in environmental health planning
Ministerial Declaration on Violence and Injury Prevention in the Americas	March 14, 2008	Recognized explicit link between key violence-related health and human rights issues (e.g., illicit traffic of small arms, violence against women and children); called for health services with focus on promotion of health, rights and specific gender and intercultural needs.
Declaration of Commitment of Port of Spain	April 19, 2009	Adopted at Fifth Summit of the Americas; commitment to protection, promotion of and respect for political and civil liberties and fundamental freedoms, especially in relation to health and environment, to improve social, economic and cultural well-being of all peoples.

Rights (ICESCR), which, as of August 2010, had been ratified by 160 parties (United Nations, 2010).

Using human rights provides a powerful authoritative basis for advocacy, cooperation and partnership-building with and among governments, international organizations and civil society partners. The Ministers of Health of the Americas have acknowledged health as a fundamental human right related to other human rights and freedoms. This acknowledgement officially recognizes human rights treaties and standards as essential instruments for restructuring health systems and for the promotion and protection of health. Table 11.1 outlines several declarations made by the Ministers of Health of the Americas over the past two decades and their significance in terms of linking health systems strengthening, human rights and improved health outcomes. This is not an exhaustive list but rather provides exemplars of the acknowledged linkage among health, human rights and health systems strengthening at the highest policy levels in our global region.

At the global level, actions were taken to build human rights accountabilities within the work of the United Nations (U.N.) organization. In answer to the U.N. Secretary General's call for integrating human rights across the entire U.N. system (United Nations, 1997), nearly all of the U.N. agencies now have explicit policies or strategies for applying rights-based approaches to their field of intervention (UNDP, 2005). The U.N. Secretary-General's "Programme for Reform" (1997) and its second phase, "An Agenda for Further Change" (2001), called upon U.N. agencies to make human rights a cross-cutting priority for the U.N. In 2003, a group of U.N. agencies, including the United Nations Population Fund (2010), committed to integrating human rights into their national development cooperation programs by adopting the aforementioned *Common Understanding* (UNESCO, 2003) on a rights-based approach.

In 2005, the WHO, as a U.N. member agency, adopted human rights as a cross-cutting theme throughout its organizational clusters. As the organization-wide focal point for human rights, the WHO Health and Human Rights Unit is housed in the Department of Ethics, Equity, Trade and Human Rights in the Cluster of Information, Evidence and Research (IER/ETH). The regional human-rights mechanism for the Americas is located within the Organization of American States (OAS) and is based upon the American Convention of Human Rights. The WHO says that it is actively strengthening its role in providing technical, intellectual and political leadership in the human rights field since this was made a cross-cutting theme (UNHR and WHO, 2008).

A number of initiatives within the WHO have been undertaken using this RBA, focusing on issues with direct impacts on health, the conditions necessary for health and the social determinants (Krug, et al., 2009; UNHR & WHO, 2008; United Nations, 2007b; WHO, 2007a, 2007b, 2010b). It is clear that health-related RBA activity has increased in intensity globally as nations work towards the health-related Millennium Development Goals, particularly for women, children and those suffering with HIV/AIDS. The Millennium Development Goals are eight international development goals that all 192 U.N. member states agreed to achieve by 2015 (WHO, 2010a).

The explicit linkages among human rights, health as a right and primary health care renewal are rarely debated in the mainstream peer-reviewed health literature. Not surprisingly, given that the first international declaration to clearly link human rights and health focused on psychiatric care, the concepts of human rights and primary health care have been linked in work on mental health in primary health care settings (McPherson & McGibbon, 2010b; Mwape et al., 2010).

From a national perspective, which is where these RBA and primary health care policy issues need closer examination, Martin (2006) discusses the legal imperative to deliver accessible primary health care within a human rights framework in England, noting that discrimination in access has always breached the norms of health ethics. Martin argues that, unlike English common law, the 1998 Human Rights Act is as much concerned with failure to protect rights as it is with positive acts in breach of rights. This imposes an obligation on English primary care trusts to monitor and adjust all access practices, policies and government documents purporting to recognize the power of the patient to choose. This emphasis on monitoring and adjustment is consistent with the need for greater accountability within an RBA framework, discussed earlier.

National health system outcomes discourse vis-à-vis current laws and policies, such as that advanced by Martin (2006), is crucial in moving the health human rights agenda forward within policy and political agendas that focus on health systems strengthening and primary health care. Although many governmental health system reforms may be well intended, an RBA to health systems and inequities analysis would force us to look at effects and outcomes *not* intentions. An RBA would support public decision-makers in identifying the indispensable deep structural changes that need to be made for health and health-relevant public services to receive the resources and education they need to reverse the rights currently being violated.

Although an RBA provides a useful legal framework and guide for public health actions, *accountability* of governments is a crucial and pivotal RBA aspect within any health systems strengthening agenda. Of primary importance in this discussion is the notion that the U.N. human rights mechanisms provide important avenues towards increasing accountability for health. Using human rights in the health sector can be a tool for strengthening laws, policies and standards of care. In some instances, as is the case in a highly developed country such as Canada, the examination of health vis-à-vis human rights should be country-led, participatory and reflective, thus supporting ownership of proposed actions. This approach sits in contrast to using an RBA within external monitoring and punitive processes.

Although some progress has been made, other points of view hold that U.N. agencies, along with many member states, have held to neoliberal policies that are responsible for the slow progress towards true health equity for all (Bryant, 2009). Neoliberalism is the policy side of the new global economic reality that essentially harmonizes the national and global economies and shifts the policy gaze from a universal national social democracy to a global agenda (Teeple, 2000). As Teeple argues, while representatives of capital (e.g., World Trade Organization, International Monetary Fund, World Bank) apply external pressure to U.N. member nations, national governments legislate neoliberal policies intended to privatize state property so as to "free capital from social forms in which it is under or open to political control and thereby turn those forms into corporate private property [to feed the global agenda]. In the end the demands of capital will have few if any official or authoritative national restraints" (81).

Fundamentally, this means that there is a diminished national budget available to apply to social programs. As McGibbon and Hallstrom discuss in Chapter 12, neoliberal policies emphasize individual responsibility and achievement and hence individualistic approaches to public policy rather than universalism and socialist ideals of equality and social rights (Bryant, 2009; Saint-Arnaud & Bernard, 2003). The current neoliberal political context clearly runs counter to a rights-based approach to health systems strengthening through primary health care.

In 2001 Braveman and colleagues argued that the 2000 World Health Report (WHO, 2000b) did not go far enough when it recommended that national health systems be assessed not only by the average health status of a country's population but also by the extent to which health varies within the population. They were concerned that the report actually undermined efforts to achieve greater equity in health within nations because it removed equity and human rights considerations from the routine measurement and reporting of health disparities within nations. A decade later, this issue is clearly still relevant as we consider health inequities and government accountability; we need to continue to question what real policy progress has been made in monitoring and operationalizing the recognized link between health and human rights.

We see some progress at global and regional levels. For example, since 1999 the Pan American Health Organization (PAHO), the WHO region covering the Americas, has promoted human rights and fundamental freedoms and expanded the use of human rights instruments from mental health to many other health contexts. As a consequence of PAHO's strategies on the dissemination of human rights norms and standards, many countries are in the process of reforming national laws and policies according to international human rights law (Peragio, 2007). However, what is not yet evident is how such high-level laws and policies are enacted, measured, enforced and reported at the country and more local levels. Further, there do not appear to be clear mechanisms to measure the ultimate impact of such measures on health inequities and population health status in the Americas. This responsibility rests with the state. Ensuring that the human rights and health worlds come together and that governments and public authorities make timely, appropriate and accessible health care available for all is a key challenge facing governments, health and other public service professionals and the human rights community.

Embedding a Rights-Based Approach in Primary Health Care

At the highest level of generality, the goal of *social policy* can be stated in terms of supporting individual well-being (Bryant, 2009). Social policy is concerned with how public social problems and issues get defined and constructed, how they are placed on political and policy agendas and how and why governments act or do not act (Heidenheimer, 1990). What difference would frameworks of a rights-based approach and primary health care make to the process and substance of social policymaking? At a minimum, policy frameworks such as these provide a way of conceptualizing the relationships between individuals and society that is consistent with emerging thinking about health and broader social policy. No explicit theory or framework comprehensively describes the goals of social policy or how social policies actually work. However, RBA and primary health care frameworks could influence the choice of broad strategic approaches regarding the pace and architecture of policy change designed to strengthen health systems. Frameworks could also help us to think about specific health and other public policy design and delivery, the construction of evaluation measures of effectiveness and decisions about "who should be doing what." These two frameworks could also be used to examine current pressures on the policy agenda as well as future policy needs and opportunities. Thus, using an RBA and primary health care as the policy frameworks could be seen as practical policy tools and imperatives to support health and public systems strengthening (as the intended social policy), which would be a means of tackling oppression and reducing health inequities (desired social outcomes).

A human rights-based approach to health systems strengthening gives us the possibility to advance policy and political agendas towards health equity. In the twenty-first century, no ministry health in the PAHO region can claim to be unaware of its duties and responsibilities to safeguard and guarantee the human and civil rights of health system users (Vásquez, 2007). With the legal right to health clearly articulated, the next logical action is to embed an RBA in primary health care policy-making and reforms. However, as we know, health systems will not automatically gravitate towards greater fairness and efficiency — there has to be a policy imperative to do so (Chan, 2009). This policy imperative exists within the health systems strengthening agenda.

What would a rights-based primary health care system look like? To answer this question, we have to consider several elements: the health system, primary health care principles and RBA principles. Table 11.2 examines these three areas and considers how each element may complement the others, with a focus on cross-sectoral collaboration. The first column lists the six building blocks of a health system, which fundamentally consists of organizations, institutions, resources and people whose primary purpose is to improve a society's health (WHO, 2010a). The second two columns outline what a rights based primary health care system would look like if internationally accepted primary health care and rights principles were integrated into the public service system. For example, embedding an RBA into primary health care policy would ensure that children were protected from the threat of violence. All appropriate legislative, administrative, social and educational measures to protect the child from all forms of physical and mental violence, injury or abuse, neglect or negligent treatment, maltreatment or exploitation, including sexual abuse, would be taken (International Convention on the Rights of the Child, UNICEF, 1989). This example speaks strongly and clearly about the need for cross-sectoral policy integration and programming.

Pushing a broad public health policy agenda using a human rights-based approach has led to much policy and health outcome success by international agencies and in many countries, such as with HIV/AIDS (Galvao, 2005; McPherson & Shamian, 2010). However, there are additional costs associated with reaching underserved populations, and there are significant challenges associated with allocating and redistributing resources against agreed priorities.

Major Issues Hindering an RBA in Primary Health Care Renewal

The still limited uptake of public sector primary health care services obviously has many roots. Historical and political contexts continue to have a major impact on the primary health care renewal culture (McPherson, Kothari, & Sibbald, 2010; McPherson & McGibbon, 2010a). A human rights approach highlights the discrimination, inequality, powerlessness and accountability failures (UNHR & WHO, 2008) that lie at the root of many social injustices and resultant ill-health. Three fundamental issues that hinder an RBA to primary health care renewal are discussed here.

Table 11.2 Application of Primary Health Care and Human Rights-Based Principles to the Six Health System Building Blocks

Health System Building Blocks (WHO, 2010a)	Primary Health Care Principles (WHO, 1978)	Human Rights-Based Approach Principles (Tomas, 2005)
Good health services and infrastructure A well-performing health workforce A well-functioning health information system Equitable access to safe essential medical products, vaccines and technologies A good health financing system Leadership and governance	Accessibility Public participation Health promotion Appropriate skills and technology Intersectoral cooperation	Participation Accountability Non-discrimination and equality Empowerment Linkages to human rights standards

1) Lack of Awareness of Rights and Responsibilities in Health

Many citizens, health professionals and public decision-makers are unaware of the linkages among human rights, primary health care service access and health inequities. There is a need to create awareness of the rights and responsibilities for health on the part of government policymakers, local service delivery agents and citizens as service users. There is an urgent need to find ways to effectively and collectively identify rights violations and to improve the system at all levels.

Fundamentally, an RBA requires recognition that a particular objective, even if presented as a political commitment or policy goal, may in fact be a binding legal obligation. Thus, an RBA requires awareness and acknowledgment of a wide range of binding legal obligations. These obligations include not only the treaties, but also the jurisprudence and other commentaries which have elaborated on treaty provisions over the past fifty years (Amnesty International & International Human Rights Network, 2005).

2) Social Value Norms Are Difficult to Shift

Incorporating an RBA in primary health care requires a shift in social value norms. The general orientation of the prevailing North American societal value system is closer to an egalitarian view of distributive justice, which advocates the equal allocation of material goods to all members of society. More consistent with primary health care and human rights-based prin-

Table 11.2 Application of Primary Health Care and Human Rights-Based Principles to the Six Health System Building Blocks
A Rights-Based Primary Health Care System Would…

- demonstrate accountability to human-rights and primary health care principles, ensure policies and implementation processes are explicitly linked to ratified human rights standards;
- develop laws and administrative procedures, practices and mechanisms that ensure the fulfillment of rights entitlements, as well as opportunities to address denials and violations;
- translate universal standards into locally determined benchmarks to measure progress;
- have a core set of functional and structural elements in place to guarantee comprehensive, universal coverage and access to equity-enhancing services over time;
- ensure access to necessary health products and technologies; optimal organization and management practices at all levels to achieve quality, efficiency, effectiveness, sustainability;
- emphasize health promotion and prevention and assure first contact care that is responsive to people's health needs, as well as the conditions necessary for health;
- be based on social justice, with a particular focus on addressing discrimination and inequality, focusing on marginalized, disadvantaged and excluded groups;
- develop governance mechanisms that empower individual and collective participation in locally owned services and that engage citizens in decisions affecting their own health;
- demonstrate leadership in working across government departments/sectors to ensure a rights-based approach to public system strengthening;
- integrate policies and cross-sectoral actions to address multiple determinants of health;
- have a sound legal, institutional and organizational foundation as well as adequate and sustainable human, financial and technological resources and information systems; and
- employ and educate human resources that are prepared to effectively practice within primary health care and human-rights-based frameworks, and in geographic areas where most needed.

ciples is the Rawlsian view, in which the "difference principle" prioritizes action favouring the most disadvantaged in society (Ridde, 2008a, 2009). The Difference Principle allows allocation that does not conform to strict equality so long as the inequality has the effect that the least advantaged in society are materially better off than they would be under strict equality (The Stanford Encyclopedia of Philosophy, 2007).

Kingdon (1995, 2001), in discussing complex public policymaking, notes that, if the problem at hand is considered too complex, there will be a tendency to find solutions to problems that are easier to resolve. This is consistent with Zahariadis (2003), who argues that the prime policy issues "thrown in garbage cans" (Cohen, March, & Zolsen, 1972) are those involving difficult changes in normative structures, such as basic value priorities in a policy.

It is very challenging from a policy and programming perspective to target excluded and marginalized people in primary health care renewal (Braveman, et al., 2001) because a focus on equity fundamentally defies social values norms. Thus we need to evaluate and strengthen the role of social norms in applying an RBA to health at all system levels. Professionals need to challenge the status quo by examining our own social values as they relate to human rights and health — especially for the most vulnerable in our society — and by using political agendas to advocate for rights-based accountability in policies, services and health outcomes.

3) Lack of Engagement of Local Communities in Renewal Planning

The Declaration of Alma-Ata (WHO, 1978) called for full participation of communities in their health services. Participation is also one of the key principles of a human rights-based approach. Canada was among the countries to have adopted the Alma-Ata thirty-three years ago, committing itself, among other things, to a human rights-based approach to health, in which "the people have the right and duty to participate individually and collectively in the planning and implementation of their health care."

Effective demand for appropriate primary health care services needs to come from the vulnerable and those who advocate for them. However, there is also a critical role for government in empowering local communities, which runs counter to a traditional defensive response from governments to demands for services. Genuine improvement in primary health care rests on involving an informed population in the planning and implementation of the overall system. This consideration is of even greater importance in resource-poor communities and nations. It is with these most vulnerable poor populations where the health impacts of the intersections of the social determinants of health are strongest (McGibbon, 2009; McPherson & McGibbon, 2010b).

A Way Forward on Health Inequities and Primary Health Care Renewal

The purpose of this chapter is not just to provide a background in the concepts of health human rights and health systems strengthening though primary health care but also to encourage the reader to think about the broader implication of what government, global health and human service agencies and communities might do in democratic societies towards reduction in oppression and in health inequities. The chapter concludes with an exploration of possible alternatives to current policy and government actions.

The arguments set forth thus far have generally represented a 20,000 foot overview of the issues at hand. The application of a rights-based approach in primary health care renewal is also contingent on the constraints and realities on the ground and on the mandates of the organizations involved. Clearly, the translation of the implications of an RBA in primary health care renewal should necessarily differ across organizational and other contexts. Although the concepts remain the same, the approach needs to be adapted to fit the context of particular communities, provinces/states, countries and global regions, recognizing that different countries have different policymaking styles (Howlet & Ramesh, 2003). The issue of translation and application variations across different contexts needs to be further explored if an RBA to primary health care is to be made transparent and the learnings made transferable.

Although mutual accountability flows among public system domains, professionals and communities, the primary responsibility for developing an RBA to primary health care renewal rests with the state due to the regulatory role of governments and their leadership role in enhancing health and broader public policy coherence. A rights-based approach needs to be seen by the state as a transformative strategy to further the goals of the state, which should, in turn, support societal well-being. Ultimately, human rights need to be seen as a useful framework to strengthen the health and broader public service system so that the goals of primary health care can be realized.

Society must explicitly recognize that the highest attainable level of health is a basic right, not a good or commodity. We all have a collective obligation to bring health and dignity to communities in need. Strong health systems and services, with anchoring primary health care foundations, are needed to ensure the human right to health. This represents a fundamental paradigm shift when talking about health system reform because the problem is not defined by availability of hospitals or physicians; rather it is defined by *a violation of the right* to those things that help keep us as healthy as possible and an associated lack of public service *accountability* for health human rights inactions and violations.

This represents a challenge to health professionals and public leaders alike. There is an urgent need to extend rights-based frameworks beyond conceptual clarity seeking and advocacy to the level of effective implementation within a primary health care policy agenda. Use of a human rights-based approach in health systems strengthening through primary health care renewal is an essential strategy, *not* an optional tool, in ensuring the human right to health.

12

Oppression and the Political Economy of Health Inequities

Elizabeth A. McGibbon and Lars K. Hallstrom

> In the popular literature generally, there has been an unwarranted tendency to equate economic development with human well-being. In fact, in the advanced capitalist countries, national wealth seems to have relatively little to do with national well-being. (Coburn, 2003, p. 349)

The perspective through which we view the nature of health is central to how we can envision paths for improving the health of individuals, families, communities and nations. Although there are notable exceptions, population health continues to be analyzed as an aggregate of the health outcomes and behaviours of individuals. Western views of the nature of the body and of health overlay this individualistic gaze. One only has to examine the health policies and systems design for acute care in the West to be reminded that we still view the human body as a system of parts, with areas of expertise and indeed hospital geography organized around these body parts. The acute care model is by far the dominant model of heath care delivery, and an individualistic approach also permeates other areas of health system delivery, such as community and public health. This is the crux of the problem — the system focus continues to be on the micro level causes of ill health, such as individual genetics, behaviour and lifestyle.

There is consistent reluctance and lack of capacity to engage in sustained and frank discussion of the systemic, structural causes of ill health. The purpose of this chapter is to add to the debate about the importance of the political economy of health. We build on previous chapters to further an understanding of the political and economic causes of ill health and hence the paths to amelioration of the suffering and deprivation at the heart of health inequities. The chapter begins with a definition and discussion of epidemiology, the dominant approach to the study of population health. We emphasize its far-reaching influence on how the genesis of ill health is understood by practitioners, researchers and policymakers and thus its impact on public policy. The origins of Navarro's (2002a, 2007a) "materialist epidemiology" are described, along with its foundations in the political economy of health.

Two case examples demonstrate the ways that neoliberal ideology has a foundational impact on the creation and maintenance of health inequities. We conclude with a discussion of tackling oppression through public policy by design.

Epidemiological Perspectives on Population Health

Epidemiology concerns itself with disease incidence, etiology and distribution. The field of epidemiology began in 1854 with John Snow's famous links between the incidence of cholera in a crowded London district and the location of city wells. Snow discovered that the highest incidence of cholera occurred around several contaminated wells. The connection between disease incidence and causation, and hence treatment, was dramatically demonstrated. Snow's work also laid the foundation for the geographic study of disease incidence. An introductory epidemiology text describes the modern-day foundations of epidemiology, including clinical questions (e.g., the accuracy of tests used to diagnose disease); variables (e.g., independent, dependent, extraneous variables); health outcomes (e.g., death, disease, disability); numbers and probability (e.g., quantitative measurement of health outcomes); and additional quantitative principles (e.g., population selection and samples) (Fletcher & Fletcher, 2005, p. 5). Epidemiology has accomplished massive population health advances in the treatment of communicable diseases, most notably in the West. Although epidemiology has historically been central in some areas of human disease management, its lack of attention to political, economic and social aspects of everyday life is increasingly problematic (McGibbon & Etowa, 2009). The fact that poverty is the main cause of poor health outcomes in Canada and globally underscores the stark limitations of conventional epidemiology. The work of social scientists and epidemiologists such as Shaw, et al. (1999) in the United Kingdom and Krieger in the United States (2001a, 2001b, 2003, 2005) demonstrates the substantial contrast between conventional epidemiology and epidemiology based in critical social science. Shaw et al.'s book, *The Widening Gap: Health Inequalities and Policy in Britain*, related mortality and morbidity statistics to poverty and housing and to the ideological foundations of public policy. The authors found that the social gradient and its longitudinal policy base were the clearest and most robust predictors, over time, of infant and child mortality and premature adult mortality. "In contemporary Britain, unequal chances of death are interwoven, in social and spatial terms, with unequal chances in life, in terms of education, employment, income, and wealth" (1999, p. 5).

The integration of critical social science with epidemiology is an increasing global trend, with its genesis in mounting concern about growing poverty rates in countries around the world, including so-called "rich countries" such as Canada and the United States. The term "social epidemiology" was first used in the *American Sociological Review* in 1950 in an article titled "The Relationship of Fetal and Infant Mortality to Residential Segregation: An Inquiry into Social Epidemiology" (cited in Krieger, 2001a). According to Krieger, this topic is as timely now as it was in 1950:

> Grappling with notions of causation, in turn, raises not only complex philosophical issues but also, in the case of social epidemiology, issues of accountability and agency: simply invoking abstract notions of "society" and disembodied "genes" will not suffice. Instead, the central question becomes: Who and what is responsible for population patterns of disease and well-being, as manifested in present, past and changing social inequalities in health. (2001a, p. 677)

Social epidemiology explicitly investigates social determinants of population distributions of health, disease and well-being, rather than treating these determinants as mere background to biomedical phenomena (Kreiger, 2001a). Vincente Navarro (2002a, 2007a: 21) extends the reach of social epidemiology to call for a materialist epidemiology which recognizes that the societal hierarchy of class relations "conditions most potently how other variables affect the population's health." Navarro and colleagues studied how race, gender and ethnicity affect health and well-being and analyzed the effects of these variables as part of a matrix of ruling relations at the core of systems of domination and subordination. In the still famous words of eighteenth-century physician and anthropologist Rudolf Virchow, "All diseases have two causes — one pathological, the other political." Materialist approaches, based in the political economy of health, provide this larger societal context for linking health outcomes across the lifespan with the structural ideologies that create and sustain oppression.

Political Economy and a Materialist Perspective on Health

Political economy analyses originated with the work of Marx and Engels, and were re-invigorated in the 1970s and 1980s (Coleman, 1982; Doyal & Pennell, 1979; McKinley, 1975) and still remain important in the twenty-first century (Navarro, 2002b; Muntaner & Lynch, 2001; Muntaner, et al., 2004). Political economy approaches are derived from two major disciplines — politics and economics. A political economy approach "interrogates economic doctrines to disclose their sociological and political premises... in sum, [it] regards economic ideas and behavior not as frameworks for analysis, but as beliefs and actions that must themselves be explained" (Mayer, 1987, p. 3). Marx was the first to describe a methodological approach to understanding the linkages among society, economics and history. Rather than viewing the field of economics as consisting of objective and quantifiable sets of measurements and models, he explored a new way to think about economics, where the politics of a nation very much influences the direction and outcomes of its economic policy.

> My inquiry led me to the conclusion that neither legal relations nor political forms could be comprehended, whether by themselves or on the basis of a so-called general development of the human mind, but that on the contrary they originate in the material conditions of life, the totality of which Hegel, following the example of English and French thinkers of the eighteenth century, embraces within the term "civil society"; that the autonomy of this civil society, however, has to be sought in political economy. (Marx, 1977 [1845])

Marx explained that in order to survive and continue existence from generation to generation, it is necessary for human beings to produce and reproduce the material requirements of life. Materialist approaches are based in his assertion that economic factors — the way people produce these necessities of life — determine the kind of politics and ideology a society can have. "The totality of these relations of production constitutes the economic structure of society, the real foundation, on which arises a legal and political superstructure and to which correspond definite forms of consciousness. The mode of production of material life conditions the general process of social, political and intellectual life" (Marx, 1977 [1845]: 175). A core aspect of a materialist approach is its foundation in interrogating how the relations of production of goods and services in a society (e.g., social structure, divisions of labour) are articulated to legal, political, religious and cultural ideology and institutions. Marx emphasized that an important aspect of this interrogation was the relationship between social class and production, namely that the ruling classes had control over the means of production. These ideas formed the historical analytic basis of much recent scholarship on political economy. Navarro (2002b); Muntaner & Lynch (2001); Muntaner, Eaton, et al., (2004); and Esping-Andersen (2002) provide detailed discussions of the ways that a political economy approach can provide solution-focused insights regarding how to tackle health inequities and their genesis in material and social deprivation.

A political economy lens is central to modern efforts to understand and tackle the "causes of the causes" of social problems, including growing inequities in health outcomes related to intersections of classism, racism and sexism, to name a few. As one might expect, materialist approaches to health care are centred on the structural determinants of health. They are called structural because "they are part of the political, economic, and social structure of society and of the culture that informs them" (Navarro, 2007a. p. 2). Political economists emphasize the role of the economic organization of society in the production and distribution of disease and burden of illness and the ways that disease and illness are framed and treated (Coburn, 2006; McGibbon, 2009). Materialist perspectives on health and health care involve public policy questions about how some groups of people persistently have worse health than others and how some countries have different kinds of health care systems and correspondingly different citizen health. Although the income inequality model, often cited as an antecedent of health inequality, acknowledges the relationship between income and health, it stops short of connecting the poor health of poor people to race and class inequality in capitalist societies (Muntaner & Lynch, 2001).

Health and Public Policy from a Structural Perspective

The makers of public policy, and health policy in particular, have a central responsibility to ensure good health for the entire population. Although all sectors and agencies should be responsible for creating conditions of optimal health and well-being of citizens, government (public authorities and their public administration) is the primary agency responsible for developing a national health policy (Navarro, 2007a). Public policy and the ideologies that underpin policy design, implementation and evaluation create the political economy of health inequities. There is considerable evidence that international, national, territorial and local health and social policies are linked to population health outcomes. Even in countries such as Canada and the U.S., listed among the "have" countries internationally, child poverty is relatively high, and in the case of the U.S., is comparable to countries in the Global South.

The structural determinants of health, although rarely listed in national health plans, are the most important in determining a population's health outcomes (Navarro, 2007a). These policies include the SDH, for example, employment and education policies, early childhood intervention and poverty reduction policies, and a social safety net that is universally accessible rather than based in a state-determined meritocracy. However, political will and hence capacity to establish these policies varies from state to state according to prevailing political ideologies. Social democratic public policies tend to lead to better health outcomes across all social classes, races, ethnicities and ages (Raphael, 2009b). In well-developed social democracies, such as Sweden, health outcomes are better for *everyone*, not only for disadvantaged, marginalized and racialized people. If the evidence is so strong that social democratic policies hold the best promise for increasing the health and well-being of citizens, why are social democratic policies not more prevalent in the West? Why is there such a gap between knowledge and action on the SDH?

Consideration of the three forms of the modern welfare state provides a context for answering these kinds of questions. The concept of the welfare state refers to the "extent to which governments or the state use their power to provide citizens with the means to live secure and satisfying lives" (Raphael, 2009a, p. 15). Using Esping-Anderson's well-known typology, the modern capitalist welfare state has three main forms: social democratic, liberal and conservative, all guided by very different structures and interests that shape institutions and policy ideologies (Esping-Andersen, 1990). Specifically, the political economies of the three forms of welfare state have central differences in the nature and extent of state intervention to provide the means necessary to meet the material and social needs of citizens. These three forms are not mutually exclusive, and varying combinations might be represented in any given set of social policies. However, overall health and social equality can nonetheless be accurately gauged as a function of a country's political economy.

Conservative political economies are based in the ideological inspiration of social stability, wage stability and social integration (Saint-Arnaud & Bernard, 2003). These principles are seen to be realized by providing benefits based on insurance schemes geared to a variety of family and occupational categories (Bryant, 2009). However, as our discussion points out, neoliberalism constitutes a somewhat paradoxical fusion of both liberal and conservative elements. We focus on social democratic and liberal welfare state practices and policies because liberalism, and specifically its modern counterpart, neoliberalism, is arguably the dominant global political ideology, while social democratic welfare states have shown the most evidence, by far, of capacity for policy intervention to address the SDH and health inequities.

In social democratic welfare states, the ideological inspiration is the reduction of poverty, inequality and unemployment. The organizing principles are universalism and the socialist ideals of equality, the social rights of all citizens, justice, freedom and solidarity (Bryant, 2009; Esping-Anderson, 2002; Saint-Arnaud & Bernard, 2003). Denmark, Finland, Norway and Sweden are the best modern exemplars of social democracies (Bryant, 2009). These states have the best health outcomes in the world, along with robust economies — thus refuting the stereotype that social democracy necessarily leads to fiscal irresponsibility. Social democratic states expend more of their national wealth for supports and services and are proactive in developing labour, family-friendly and gender-equity supporting policies (Raphael, 2009a). The emphasis is thus on establishing policies that increase public capacity for collective action.

In contrast, liberal welfare states are based in the ideology of liberty, with relatively minimum government intervention and a focus on benefits available only through means testing rather than universal availability. The emphasis is on individual responsibility and individual achievement, and hence individualistic approaches to public policy. Liberal welfare strategies illustrate the difference between social insurance programs, which are available to all citizens, and social assistance, which is available only to those who are destitute or in danger of becoming destitute. "Within liberal welfare states, liberty, and its close neighbor, self-determination, become available only to a narrow band of the population — those who have sufficient financial resources and cultural capital to define their own living conditions" (Raphael & Curry-Stephens, 2009, p. 366). Liberal welfare states also promote minimal government intervention in the marketplace, a framework that allows increasing privatization of health care delivery. Examples of liberal welfare states are Canada, the United States, the United Kingdom and Ireland (Bryant, 2009).

The modern iteration of the liberal welfare state is neoliberalism. Neoliberal social and economic policies have increasingly dominated public policy in Canada and elsewhere (Raphael & Bryant, 2006b). "Neoliberalism is the belief that that the marketplace should be the arbiter of how economic and other resources are distributed" (Raphael, 2009a, p. 32). Neoliberalism began in the 1980s in the U.S. and the U.K. with the Reagan and Thatcher eras respectively and the restructuring of world capitalism. Navarro (2007b), described the following tenets of neoliberalism: 1) the state needs to reduce its interventionism in economic and social activities; 2) labour and financial markets need to be deregulated in order to liberate the enormous creative energy of the markets; and 3) commerce and investments need to be stimulated by eliminating borders and barriers to allow for the full mobility of labour, financial capital, goods and services. Overbeek and van der Pijl (1993: xi) state that neoliberalism is thus to be understood as a transnational phenomenon rather than as a series of unrelated national developments.

It is therefore possible to see that while neoliberalism can be identified at the policymaking level through its emphasis on open markets and the limited role of the state, there is an underlying ideology at play. This ideology is centred in the liberal tradition of the individual and perhaps as well elements of "American exceptionalism," in which the economic sphere is held separate from the social and the political, thus removing many of the linkages between economic and political life (see, for example, Hochschild 1981; Lipset 1996). Stemming from the economic and political crisis of capitalism in the 1970s, a phase Overbeek and van der Pijl (1993) refer to as characterized by corporate liberalism, neoliberalism can be understood as an essentially successful attempt to reformulate the conditions under which the global pursuit and accumulation of capital took place. However, contrary to the theoretical foundations of neoliberalism and the political rhetoric of political leaders exemplifying the "new right," such as Reagan and Thatcher, this attempt was only successful for specific groups, creating, as Petras and

Vieux (1992) call it, the "stolen decade" for Latin America. The success of neoliberalism can therefore be assessed on two levels: 1) its capacity to re-formulate the dominant paradigm for capital accumulation; and 2) its ability to provide a better means of capital accumulation.

Understood as an ideological disposition toward creating a legitimate and alternative form of capital accumulation, neoliberalism has relied not only on the view that individuals can best judge their needs (Held 1989), neces-sarily limiting the importance of the state, but also on creating a "politics of support" (Gamble, 1988) through a neoconservative emphasis on "moral conservatism, xenophobia, law-and-order, the family" (Overbeek and van der Pijl, 1993, p. 15). As a result, neoliberalism, the dominant ideology of the late twentieth century, has become premised on democratic support, anti-communism/socialism and the primacy of the free-market or *laissez-faire* society, creating, as Zamora points out (in Rosen & McFayden (1995), a cult(ure) of capitalism, unconstrained by any factors except for the limits created by physical forms of capital.

Neoliberalism then may be identified as the new conception/construc-tion of capital accumulation following the 1970s, built at the practical level on a somewhat paradoxical fusion of both liberal and conservative elements (Held, 1989). From the liberal perspective, neoliberalism emphasizes the im-portance of individual freedom of choice, minimal government intervention and the *laissez-faire* society. However, in "rolling back the state" on the basis of such grounds, governments have focused not only on policies to ensure conditions for the individual pursuit of interests but also on the establish-ment of a secure environment for the pursuit of prosperity (capital). As a consequence, neoliberalism is a strategy to limit the scope of the state, while simultaneously demanding strong government, hierarchy, discipline and a general increase in the capacity of the state to ensure political stability (Held 1989; Overbeek & van der Pijl 1993).

As a result of this strategy, the word *liberal* has become perhaps the most fashionable phrase of the Third Wave of democratization, implying, through an emphasis on free markets, a direct contrast to the controls and central plan-ning of the Soviet Union. When prefixed with the *neo*, it becomes a descriptor of both this new strategy and the new policies of capital accumulation: free trade, privatization of public activity, deregulation, limits and reductions in social spending and a reliance on the market to solve social problems, despite evidence of the inability of economic mechanisms to do so (Rosen & McFayden, 1995; Eckersley, 1995). It is difficult to imagine the complexity of how these concepts (e.g., neoliberalism, liberal and conservative thinking, capitalism and states' economic ideologies) are related to health and public policy. However, SDH-related injustice and suffering unfold in the practical, real world. The following examples illustrate some of the contrasting policy implications between neoliberal and materialist approaches to public policy and their impact on ways of thinking about the constituents of health and well being.

Policy Example: A Public Health Approach to Chronic Disease
Policy interventions for reducing chronic disease illustrate some of the differences between neoliberal and materialist political economies. Obesity, diabetes and heart disease are all positively correlated with poverty. Despite the robust correlation between chronic diseases and the SDH, public policy approaches to reducing chronic disease continue to focus largely on individualistic solutions, thus delaying much-needed systemic intervention. The following example is based in a 2010 Ontario Public Health Association (OPHA, 2010) document which provided four public health activities, along with examples (see columns one and two in Table 12.1). We have added a third column, "Structural Policy Approach," to provide a comparison between neoliberal, and hence individualistic, approaches and structural approaches.

As Table 12.1 attests, neoliberal policy approaches to chronic disease demonstrate serious limitations, including a strong emphasis on individuals, families and communities as the unit of analysis, and a lack of capacity or an unwillingness to tackle structural, SDH approaches to prevention of chronic disease.

Policy Example: Environmental Toxins, Corporate Profit and Health
Chapter 1 details some of the mechanisms that drive oppressive processes and practices against marginalized peoples and groups. There is a synergy with these oppressive processes and mechanisms such as the increasing corporatization of natural and human resources, including its disastrous impacts on health across generations. The following environmental toxin examples underscore the neoliberal primacy of the market. In local and international realms, the health implications of market-driven environmental ravages are increasingly being scrutinized. Geographers and others have documented the significant health impacts of chronic exposure to industrial waste. These examples illustrate the gravity of exposure to industrial toxins on human health and their origins in corporate profit. As Chernomas and Hudson (2009) so clearly point out, the health of all human peoples, and indeed all life on the planet, is in peril as a result of economic policies that reinforce the primacy of profit over health and well-being. For example, resting on the phosphate industry's gypsum piles are highly acidic wastewater ponds littered with toxic contaminants, including fluoride, arsenic, cadmium, chromium, lead, mercury and the decay-products of uranium. When leaked into the environment, this poisonous high-volume cocktail wreaks havoc on waterways, watersheds and fish populations (Connett, 2003).

Table 12.1 Neoliberal and Structural Policy Approaches to Reducing Chronic Disease		
Public Health Activity*	**Neoliberal Policy Approaches***	**Structural (Materialist) Policy Approaches**
Population health assessment	Understanding the characteristics of a specific community and what must be done to effectively support the health of that community.	Understanding the historical antecedents and current dynamics of the relationships among public policy, chronic disease and policy-based social and material deprivation in a specific community.
Example	Forming a workplace health committee to assess opportunities for healthy eating and to create a workplace policy for access to nutritional food.	Linking the Longitudinal First Nations Community Health Survey (2007) with colonial and imperial policies and their current impact on capacity for healthy eating among Indigenous peoples.
Surveillance and monitoring	Assessing the incidence of chronic disease and the related risk behaviours and conditions in specific communities.	Assessing the incidence of chronic physical and mental health problems in specific communities, with emphasis on the context of risk-producing oppressive social and environmental conditions (e.g., policy-created poverty).
Example	Ongoing surveys of the public to determine levels of physical activity over time.	Establishing longitudinal health report cards that track social safety net erosion with incidence of chronic disease across geography, income, education, gender, ethnicity, race, disability and so on.

Table 12.1 Neoliberal and Structural Policy Approaches to Reducing Chronic Disease		
Health promotion	Working with government and stakeholders to build community capacity to speak out for healthy policies and supportive environments that address health issues.	Developing policy-entrenched mechanisms to provide the material and social conditions for increasing the political action capacities of citizens (e.g. eradication of poverty and unemployment).
Example	Training parents in planning, shopping for and preparing food; "walking school bus"; legislation requiring restaurants to post nutritional content on menus.	Creating a robust national network of federally funded community health centres that follow the principles of the Alma Ata Declaration to mobilize parents for social action to decrease child health inequities.
Health protection	Enforcing health protection laws and minimizing health hazards that are known to have an impact on the incidence of chronic diseases.	Establishing and enforcing legal mechanisms to decrease and halt the production of market-driven environmental toxins.
Example	Eliminating exposure to secondhand smoke.	Geographic linking of chronic health conditions such as asthma and prostate cancer to pollutants listed in the National Pollution Release Inventory (see Figures 12.1, 12.2).

Source for Public Health Activity and examples in Neoliberal column: Ontario Public Health Association 2010: 4.

In Canada, living near pesticide production factories is positively correlated with breast and prostate cancer (Gardner, 2008), and fluorine pollution related to phosphate fertilizer in the soil is positively correlated with the death of grazing farm animals (Connett, 2003). Figures 12.1 to 12.4 illustrate these direct correlations, as well as the strong correlation between living near a power generation plant and developing colon and prostate cancer (Gardner, 2008). The bars depict the cancer rate in the Districy Health Authority or Region that contains the area indicated (e.g. Brandon, Lingan). Due to confidentiality reasons, information is only available for areas with more than five incidences of cancer.

The Endocrine Society (Diamanti-Kandarakis, et al., 2009), an international organization of endocrine scientists, published its first Scientific Statement in 2009 regarding endocrine-disrupting chemicals (EDCs). EDCs are substances in our environment, food and consumer products that interfere with hormone biosynthesis and metabolism. The result is a deviation from normal control over human reproduction (Diamanti-Kandarakis, et al.). EDCs are found in pesticides, industrial chemicals, plastics and plasticizers, fuels and many other chemicals that are in widespread industrial use. The Society presented evidence that endocrine disrupters have effects on male and female reproduction, breast development and breast cancer, prostate cancer, neurological and cardiovascular endocrinology and thyroid metabolism and obesity. "Results from animal models, human clinical observations, and epi-

Figure 12.1 Prostate Cancer Rate vs. Pesticide and Fertilizer Use: Variation From Case Control (Canadian Average)

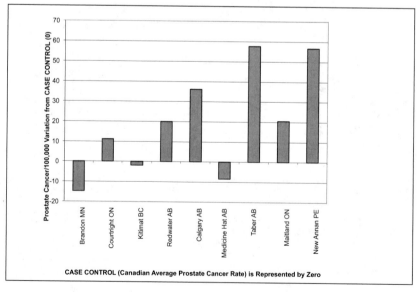

Figure 12.2 Male Colon Cancer Rate vs. Power Generation Plant: Variation from Case Control (Canadian Average)

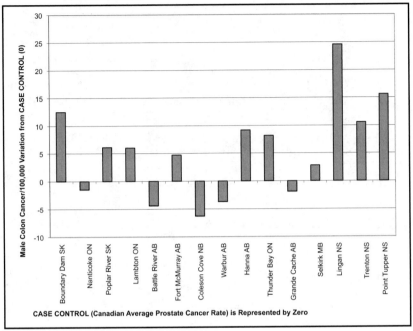

demiological studies converge to implicate EDCs as a significant concern to public health" (p. 293). Despite the undisputed science of these conclusions, in Canada there has been little sustained public health attention to these disturbing findings.

A similar pattern of the inability to sustain public health scrutiny of the profoundly negative effects of corporate profit on health and the environment may be seen in the well-known proliferation of the tar sands in Alberta. Oil sands are found in about seventy countries, and Alberta is home to the largest oil sands deposits. When oil is processed, the waste water and solids are discharged into vast tailings ponds at the rate of 1.8 billion litres per day, covering more than 130 square kilometres in northern Alberta (Dyer & Woynillowicz, 2008; Tenenbaum, 2009). The oil company Syncrude's tailings ponds, at 540 million cubic metres in volume, form one of the world's largest dams, second only to China's Three Gorges Dam. Statistically significant increases in cancers of the blood and lymphatic system, bilary tract and soft tissue were found in individuals, including many Aboriginal families, living in Fort Chipewyan, which lies in a depositional basin of tar ponds byproducts. Women in the area were found to have a 3.5 times higher risk of lung cancer (Timoney, 2007). The incidence of a rare form of bilary duct cancer

Figure 12.3 Breast Cancer Rate vs. Pesticide and Fertilizer Factories: Variation From Case Control (Canadian Average)

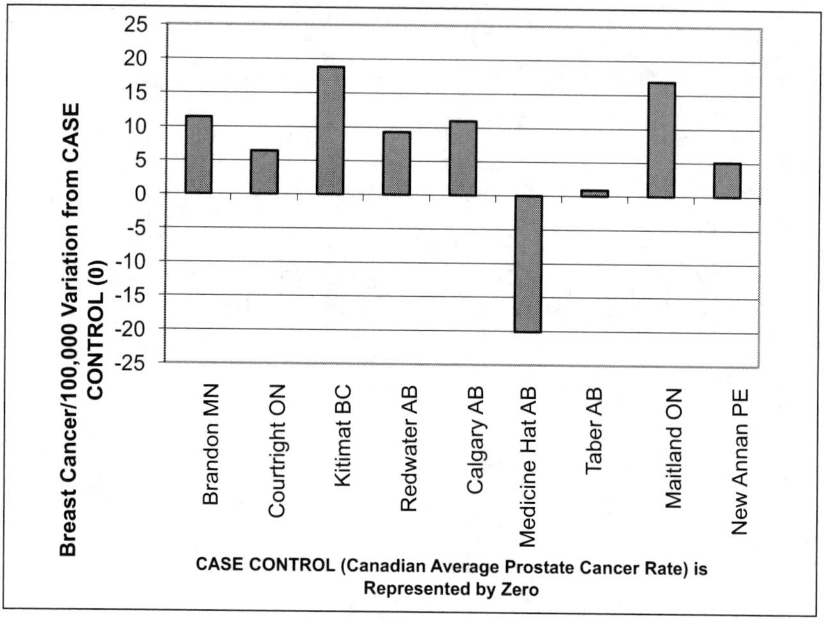

has steadily increased over the past thirty years in Alberta, and rates are two to three times higher in First Nations communities, when compared with non-First Nations populations (Tenenbaum, 2009).

In Alberta, "the feverish expansion of oil sands development is based on the untested assumption that mined landscapes can be recovered to something close to the pre-development ecosystem after mining is complete. Reclamation is the final step that mining companies are required to complete before mine closure" (Dyer & Woynillowicz, 2008, p. 1). To date, the Government of Alberta has certified as reclaimed land only 0.2 percent of the total land base disturbed by mines. This percentage does not include tailings that companies propose to incorporate into the reclaimed landscape — a fantastically erroneous proposition, given that the toxic tailing lakes are the largest human-made structures in the world and can be seen from space (Hatch & Price, 2008). A development with significant human, environmental, social and economic costs, the tar sands provides a disturbing modern instance of the ways that the fluidity of global capital and the pursuit of profit can trigger direct and indirect health impacts which are wide-ranging and distributed unequally across the population.

The continued failure of the province of Alberta to adopt and implement a wetlands policy is another example. At first glance, it might seem strange to link water and water policy directly to health. However, as both the cases

Figure 12.4 Prostate Cancer Rate vs. Power Generation Plant: Variation from Case Control
(National Average)

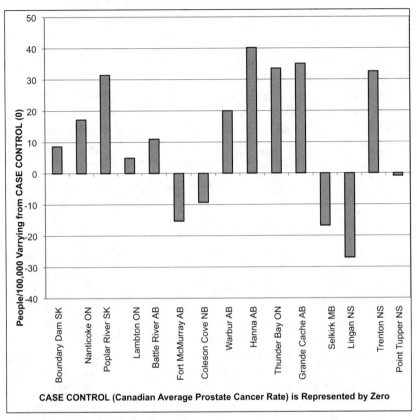

noted above, water provides more than a direct source of human health, and potentially, illness via contamination. In the case of northern Alberta, while wetlands are recognized by the province as providing major ecological, cultural and filtering (i.e., public health) benefits, the Wetland Policy in Alberta, as part of the Water for Life strategy, has been blocked and delayed since 2008, and as of summer 2010, the policy had yet to be adopted. This policy is an attempt to redress the significant loss of wetlands and wetland functionality due to both agricultural, and more recently industrial, development. In addition to the estimated 60 percent loss of wetlands in the south of the province, 23,000 hectares may be impacted by petroleum development in the north, specifically due to oil sands development.

Such petroleum development has already played a role in delaying the adoption of the Wetland Policy, for example, through formal objections to some of its requirements Both the Alberta Chamber of Resources and the Association of Petroleum Producers objected to the term "will" in sections of the policy concerned with mitigation and compensation, on the grounds that such a requirement would impede "sustainable development." There are obvious costs to the adoption of the policy, given the nature and location of northern petroleum development, with estimates ranging from $100 million to over $1 billion in mitigation costs for some projects. More importantly, however, are the health implications of this policy domain. Not only have mitigation sites in the U.S. impacted the filtration capacity of wetlands, but this capacity is not distributed equally or equitably across populations. From a political economy perspective, these massive public health concerns (e.g., tar sands, toxic watersheds) stem from unregulated capital accumulation and its origins in the increasing foothold of neoliberal public policies. Persistent government and public health system neglect of the human and ecosystem consequences of this accumulation remain one of the most pressing ethical concerns of our time.

Policy Implications for Reducing Health Inequities

Significant ink has been spilled in recent years about the importance of reducing health inequities and addressing some of the structural drivers of those inequities. Examples include the WHO Commission on the Social Determinants of Health (CSDH, 2008), the Canadian Reference Group on the SDH (Public Health Agency of Canada, 2007) and even the 2008 Canadian Heart Health Strategy and Action Plan (Smith, 2009). In addition, some attention has been given to the importance of explicitly linking public policy and policy analysis to multi-domain and intersectoral action, for example, the Canadian contribution to the Inter-Sectoral Action element of the WHO Commission on the SDH. However, as this chapter demonstrates, there are significant ideological and institutional/structural factors that limit the possibilities of health policy reform in this area (Atkinson 2002; Banting, 2005; Hess 2004). In particular, it is important to realize that not only are such factors extremely resistant to reform (in fact, political institutions and public policies are often designed to be very difficult to change) but also that such change is complicated by issues of culture, values and political capital that these changes may require. As a result, and as Banting (2005) and others have noted (Howlett & Ramesh, 2003), questions of political will, culture and the incorporation of values into public policy become paramount.

At the heart of the shift toward the neoliberal welfare state lies a much more fundamental political and cultural question: equality. As most scholars of neoliberalism and globalization attest, much of the ideological and practical impetus behind the neoliberal shift can be traced back to elements of both conservative Western philosophy and to some of the underlying principals found in the U.S. Specifically, while Canada, the U.K. and the U.S. have all promoted variants of the neoliberal welfare state via the "Third Way" of U.S.

President Clinton and British Prime Minister Tony Blair, the underlying premise and for many, driver of neoliberalism, lies in US political culture and policies and the political values which have shaped both domestic and international policies (Fukuyama 1996; Hochschild 1981; Gill 1993). In the context of health inequities, it is important to consider whether these American political foundations are becoming more prevalent in the Canadian public and in provincial and federal public policies, despite ever-mounting evidence about the SDH, racial and income-based inequalities and the widening gap between the "haves" and the "have nots," and to borrow a term from former President George Bush, the "have mores."

The shift to, and resilience of, neoliberalism may be partially explained by Hochschild's (1981) postulation that the American cultural orientation toward equality can be understood on two axes: 1) equality (of condition or of opportunity) and 2) domain (social, political or economic). Hochschild found that while there are numerous theoretical and philosophical arguments for the redistribution of wealth in a democracy, the American experience does not reflect this probability. Although Americans may view political and social equality from the standpoint of equality of condition, this expectation does not hold for the economic domain, the area that is crucially relevant for decreasing health and social inequities; disparities in economic status remain the strongest predictor of health inequities. At best, and in keeping with the American Creed (Lipset, 1996), citizens might expect that the conditions exist in order to support economic *opportunity*.

While Lipset (1996) argues that there are significant cultural or value differences between Canada and the United States, others note the changes in values that have taken place over the past thirty years in both countries. The germane question here is whether or not the Canadian public, and Canadian public policy, have come to reflect something more akin to Hochschild's axes of equality and domain, which problematizes not only the importance of economic equality and income redistribution but also health and health equity. Although issues of wait times and the delivery of health services continue to dominate the health policy domain, it is increasingly important to articulate the ideological and cultural values that drive such debates, as well as the need for different approaches to health policy that can accommodate, and if necessary, challenge those values. In the final section of this chapter, we present some possibilities that may inform thinking about Canadian and provincial health policy, and in particular emphasize the need for policy thinking that can: (a) recognize and articulate the values that underlie public policy; (b) accept and work within contexts of complexity, variability and sensitivity; and (c) permit both integrated and integrative approaches toward public policy that address the increasingly recognized linkages between health and other policy domains, often well outside the health policy field.

Health Policy by Design

Although the concept of health policy design has expanded and become increasingly used in fields as diverse as rural development, architecture and engineering, it presents particular challenges and opportunities for public policy. Design presents an opportunity not only to acknowledge and incorporate the values currently within health policy. It also permits a degree of context sensitivity, the application and use of selected tools and a focus on the possibility of change as a result of human agency (Bobrow & Dryzek 1987).

Policy design, particularly in the context of health policy, may also be a beneficial tool because of the very nature of health policy and the powerful, yet often under-recognized, influence of neoliberalism and the biomedical model. In particular, the promise of health policy design lies in its potential to recognize, articulate and critique the multiple and often conflicting values behind health policy. For example, while the value of "being healthy" may not be challenged, redistributive or equity-based values tend to prompt more debate. Importantly, not only can policy design be aware of, or include, the values present in Canadian society, but it also has the potential to include a process or procedures to articulate, critique and ultimately move toward consensus on those values driving public policy. This capacity is particularly important for health policy; as this entire chapter attests, public policy, and health policy in particular, is imbued with highly political, and therefore contestable, ideological positions. The opportunity to identify, acknowledge and debate the role of these ideologies and the values behind them, is a critical element to the ongoing development of health policy discourse.

In addition to the potential benefit of incorporating and expanding values into public policy and policy analysis, health policy design bears the possibility of being able to adapt to, and take account of, issues of complexity, context, variability and feedback. As a result, and as other more anthropologically and culturally informed analyses of public policy have demonstrated (see Guehlstorf & Hallstrom, 2005), what emerges is a model for public policy and policy analysis that is much more recursive, such that "the latter stages can both advance upon and reopen earlier phases" (Bobrow & Dryzek, 1987). It offers both an opportunity for critical examination and the possibility of synthesis. In the context of a shift toward neoliberalism, individualism and market-driven health care, a recursive model opens up the often-implicit assumptions, actions and effects of the values driving health policy in Canada. Such an approach holds great promise for the reduction of health inequities.

Perhaps even more importantly, health policy by design has the potential to spark a greater realization of how integrated the effects of public policies and interventions can be. As this chapter demonstrates, while health and well-being are often assumed, both ideologically and medically, to be individual-based, the reality is that individual, community and population health and well-being are all dependent upon numerous and interlinked social, economic, political and ecological factors. Although policy by design does not provide an explicit model for actively integrating public policy domains, as has been undertaken to a greater degree in the European Union, it does permit critical reflection and the greater possibility of linking non-health policy such as employment, infrastructure, urban planning, environment and education, to name only a few, to a more broadly defined form of health policy.

Such integration, which is inherently complex and dynamic, requires an explicit statement and assessment of the values underlying the process, purpose and method of integration. For example, the European Coal and Steel Consortium (the precursor of the European Union), originally began integration not just as an economic process to reduce transaction costs of trade, but as a peacekeeping and containment strategy to limit the military capacity of postwar Germany. In a similar vein, the benefits of health policy by design may allow policymakers and analysts to move beyond the more conventional tools of health impact assessment as they consider integration, or the possibilities of intersectoral action, as termed by the WHO. Although both environmental and health impact assessments are important steps in the consideration of the multiple and often unintended consequences of public policy, they rarely take into account the values, principles or political goals underlying policy. Instead, they are concerned with effect. However, rather than asking what the potential or previous effects of a policy might be on human health and well-being, approaching health policy from a design perspective can prompt critical analysis and examination of the economic, social and political values underlying non-health policy, as well as recognizing the importance of community engagement, socio-cultural context and variability on the basis of geographic, cultural, political, institutional and other distinctions.

Conclusions

Ultimately, there is no question that health policy, like most other policy domains, is an inherently political field (Stone 1997). However, while historically, Canadians have focused on health care, infrastructure and the provision of health services, it is increasingly important from an economic, political and environmental standpoint to consider health policy not only from the standpoint of social and economic equality and potentially even redistribution, but also with the realization, as Marmot (2008) points out, that the costs of so many human activities, whether economic, environmental or political, are not borne equally. As so many critical and neo-Marxist scholars have noted, those least able to absorb these costs typically are those who must bear them — a political consideration surely worthy of Canadian elected officials, policymakers and the general public.

13

Health as Human Right

Challenges and Supports for Accountability

Elizabeth A. McGibbon & Maureen Shebib

> Disparities in health status among different population groups
> are unjust and inequitable because they result from preventable,
> avoidable, systemic conditions and policies based on imbalances in
> political power. Without a perspective grounded in values of social
> justice, approaches to inequities in health will likely aim at symptoms,
> continuing to rely on cures, treatments or individual interventions
> rather than transforming institutions that cause health inequities.
> (Hofrichter, 2003, p. 12)

Chapter 11 discusses the international evolution of human rights and a
rights-based approach primary health care renewal, This chapter critically
presents key contexts and possibilities regarding the justiciability of health
as a human right, with an emphasis on the Canadian context. We begin with
a discussion of core concepts of human rights, particularly the evolution of
health as a human right, including challenges in definition and jurisprudence.
An individual rights perspective is briefly described and contrasted with the
increasing global emphasis on the collective rights of equity-seeking groups.
Although a complex network of national and international instruments, covenants and treaties has been developed to support human rights, including
health as a human right, we provide examples of how the justiciability of these
rights remains highly problematic. If individuals think that their rights have
been violated, they must undertake and finance the onerous task of proving
that a wrongdoing has occurred. The collective rights of groups of people,
such as Indigenous peoples, are even more difficult to garner, since violation
of these rights originate in systemic oppression based on identities such as
race, ethnicity and national origin. Finally, we describe some practical ways
to move forward in supporting states to monitor and improve performance
in upholding the right to health, delineating a rights-based health report
card for Canadian jurisdictions (McGibbon, Etowa, & McPherson, 2008b).
The chapter concludes with a discussion of economic globalization and its
barriers to upholding the right to health.

Health as a Human Right: Core Concepts

A rights perspective on health care re-frames healthy population outcomes as legally enforceable entitlements, rather than a desired, but not always achievable, goal. For example, an equity-based human rights perspective on health care would create the framework for courts and tribunals to recalibrate their legal interpretations of the *Canadian Charter of Rights and Freedoms*, (hereafter referred to as the *Charter*) and federal, provincial and territorial human rights legislation. Short of reform to human rights legislation, an equity-based interpretation and application of these instruments is required to move equitable health care and equitable health outcomes from the margins to the centre — from a possibility to a norm.

The social movement to link health and human rights is relatively recent. The United Nations implemented the first worldwide public health and human rights strategy in the 1980s, through its global AIDS program. World Health Organization (WHO) initiatives in the 1990s, based on the U.N. Universal Declaration of Human Rights (U.N., 1948), brought health and human rights together in international law (Gruskin, Mills, & Tarantala, 2007; McGibbon & Etowa, 2009). Decades earlier, during the challenge of the Jim Crow laws, which legalized the dehumanization of African-Americans, leaders in the civil rights movement in the United States linked civil rights with the right to health care, based on the lack of access to basic health care for African-American people. The successful challenge of these laws led to the creation of a civil rights report card, which detailed the results of human rights violations in the health care system (Smith, 1998, 2005a). This direct link between human rights and health care was one of the earliest strategies to address health inequities through enforcement of equitable health care treatment.

Discussions of the right to health are fraught with philosophical and definitional complexities, not the least of which is the debate about the right to health versus the right to healthiness. Toebes (1999a), in her volume *The Right to Health as a Human Right in International Law,* details some of these complexities, particularly the problems of definition and conceptual clarity regarding the normative content of the right to health and implementation practice, including reporting procedures and justiciability of the right. Toebes notes that the notion of "health" is highly subjective and that the right to "health care" and "health protection" are more realistic. As detailed in this chapter, the right to health is firmly entrenched in numerous international human rights instruments. Most treaty provisions stipulate a right to the highest attainable standard of physical and mental health, including government commitments regarding the preconditions for health, such as occupational and environmental health (Toebes, 1999a). In view of these instruments, for Toebes, it becomes clear that the problem with the right to health is not so much a lack of codification but rather an absence of consistent implementation practice through reporting procedures, and before judicial and quasi-judicial bodies, as well as lack of conceptual clarity. These problems are interrelated: a lack of understanding of the meaning and the scope of a right makes it difficult to implement, and the absence of a frequent practice of implementation in turn hampers the possibility of obtaining a greater understanding of its meaning and scope. (662)

For the purposes of discussion in this chapter, the right to health embraces the following two areas: 1) elements related to health care; and 2) elements concerning the underlying preconditions for health, including a healthy environment, safe drinking water and adequate sanitation, occupational health and access to health information (Toebes, 1999a).

Historically, the field of health and human rights has focused on the state's obligation to individual citizens, with specification of groups of people who have been historically disadvantaged in areas such as prospects for education and employment, economic stability, land ownership, physical and mental health safety and security, and a host of other areas where there is robust evidence of the persistent impact of systemic oppression. Here we define equity-seeking groups as those specified in *Charter*-enumerated non-discrimination grounds, as per section 15(1): race, national or ethnic origin, colour, religion, sex, age or mental or physical disability, and non-enumerated grounds such as sexual orientation. The Supreme Court of Canada has stated that the enumerated list is not exhaustive, and one of the first examples of judicial expansion of the enumerated grounds was its declaration that citizenship was an analogous ground deserving protection by section 15(1) (*Andrews v. Law Society of British Columbia*, 1989, CanLII 2 (S.C.C.), p. 4).

Although individual rights are foundational for a just society, there is increasing concern about how human rights, as prescribed in state legislation and numerous international covenants and treaties, can encompass systemic oppression. Hence, there are three key areas that urgently need to be debated and analyzed in terms of a rights-based approach to health including accountability mechanisms. First, how can these individual and group rights, as laid out in the various human rights instruments, be upheld? Second, how can a human rights approach support justice for collectives of oppressed peoples? For example, as Henry, Tator, Mattis and Rees (2000: 343) point out, "The liberal discourses of multiculturalism, rights, and equality are largely framed on a passive model of state intervention that ignores collective or group rights based on race." Third, where is human rights accountability to be found within the context of economic globalization? The following section explores the first two areas, with an emphasis on the justiciability of human rights instruments in the case of individual and group complaints, and concludes with an example of a human rights-based health report card as a mechanism to uphold the right to health care access and health protection of collectives of oppressed people.

Canadian Human Rights Instruments and the Right to Health

The *Charter* is part of the Constitution of Canada. Under Section 32, it applies to all matters within the authority of federal, provincial and territorial governments. Section 15(1) sets out Canadians' right to equality and establishes that "every individual is equal before and under the law and has the right to the equal protection and equal benefit of the law without discrimination." As noted earlier, this section explicitly identifies equity-seeking groups. Additionally, section 15(2) of the *Charter* permits affirmative action programs, which are laws or programs aimed at ameliorating the conditions of disadvantaged groups, including those groups set out in s. 15(1). In 1989 the Supreme Court defined discrimination under section 15 of the *Charter* as follows:

> Discrimination is a distinction which, whether intentional or not, but based on grounds relating to personal characteristics of the individual or group, has an effect which imposes disadvantages not imposed upon others or which withholds or limits access to advantages available to other members of society. (*Andrews v. Law Society of British Columbia*, 1989, 1 S.C.R. 143)

This section thus specifies treatment without discrimination. The words "without discrimination" require more than a mere finding of distinction between the treatment of groups or individuals. These words are a form of qualifier built into s. 15 itself and limit those distinctions which are forbidden by the section to those which involve prejudice or disadvantage. Given that not all distinctions and differentiations created by law are discriminatory, a complainant under s. 15(1) must show not only that she or he is not receiving equal treatment before and under the law, or that the law has a differential impact on her or him in the protection or benefit of the law, but they must also show that the law is discriminatory (*Andrews v. Law Society of British Columbia*, 1989, 1 S.C.R. 143). However, section 15 is subject to section 1 of the *Charter*, which states that the Charter guarantees rights and freedoms, with the caveat that rights are guaranteed only to such reasonable limits prescribed by law as can be demonstrably justified in a free and democratic society. For example, this distinction is at the heart of numerous debates involving areas such as Charter rights to an individual's freedom of speech in the context of what some define as hate speech. Holocaust denial remains a key example of the tensions between s. 1 of the *Charter* (i.e., freedom of speech) and s. 15 (right to non-discrimination). Clearly, societal contexts (i.e., cultural, political, ideological) heavily influence judicial decision-making, as demonstrated by the gradual legal acknowledgement of Indigenous treaty rights in Canada and elsewhere.

Judicial determinations with respect to discrimination under the *Charter* require a two-step analysis. The first step is to determine whether or not an infringement of a guaranteed right has occurred. The burden of proof rests on the citizen to establish that the infringement has occurred. As detailed later in this chapter, there are inherent flaws, often prohibitive, in requiring a citizen to bear this burden. The second step is to determine whether, if there has been an infringement, it can be justified under section 1. Under s. 1, the state is responsible for proving this infringement (*Andrews v. Law Society of British Columbia*, 1989, 1 S.C.R. 143). Governments often justify the infringement on the grounds that it would be too costly to eliminate. As previously stated, decisions are always made within prevailing societal contexts.

Challenges brought under section 15(1) of the *Charter* regarding discriminatory/social inequities have led to the advancement of equity in a number of areas. An example related to the right to access to health care is found in the case *Eldridge v. British Columbia (Attorney General*, 1997, CanLII 327 (S.C.C.)). In *Eldridge*, deaf individuals, who generally communicate using sign language, made the claim under s. 15(1) that they were being discriminated against because they were not provided with sign language interpretation services when accessing medical services provided by the Province of British Columbia. The Supreme Court ruled that deaf people were being denied their rights to equitable treatment and accordingly ordered that hospitals must provide sign language interpreters.

However, s. 15(1) of the *Charter* enables governments to argue that some forms of discrimination or inequities can be justified. For example, s. 15(1) would allow discrimination, such as barriers or limits to equitable health care, if the responding government can show that the inequity can be "demonstrably justified in a free and democratic society." This allowance of discrimination is achieved primarily through arguing a prohibitive financial burden if the government department were to be compelled to provide the service in question. As the example of provision of interpreters attests, this can be successfully challenged. The Supreme Court has by and large tended toward liberal interpretations of s. 15 and has held governments to a high standard regarding their attempts to use s. 1 to avoid the provision of equity. If the federal government's future Supreme Court appointments result in a more conservative thinking bench, s. 15 rights may undergo slippage, with s. 1 defences gaining more ground (i.e., where the Supreme Court agrees that discrimination has taken place but rejects corrective action on the grounds of the prohibitive cost of eliminating the discrimination).

In addition to *Charter*-based human rights protections, there are federal, provincial and territorial human rights statutes. These statutes are considered to be quasi-constitutional, trumping most other federal and provincial laws where the latter are in conflict with human rights legislation. On their face, these instruments provide a legal and social policy basis for civil society pressure to remove barriers to the right to health, including barriers to health care access. All human rights statutes afford protection, express or implied, to all grounds of discrimination set out therein, such as race, gender, disability, etc. However, none explicitly recognize poverty and related challenges facing women and men, for example, living in rural communities with limited health care services and transportation. In order to question the constitutionality of barriers to full citizen rights, such as persistent family poverty, citizens must launch a legal challenge, a relatively rare and arduous process. Since there is no direct access to the Supreme Court, the challenge must start in a provincial court, and lower court rulings must be appealed to the Supreme Court. Should citizens succeed in lower courts, the government or institutional respondent will almost certainly appeal. It can take years and an enormous amount of money before a case reaches the Supreme Court.

Furthermore, the principles applied under human rights statutes support both the rights defined in the *Charter* (i.e., rights of equity seeking groups) and its s. 1 limitations (i.e., only to such reasonable limits prescribed by law as can be justified in a free and democratic society). Thus, the use of federal and provincial human rights legislation by individual and group complainants is likewise hamstrung by government counter-arguments under or akin to s. 1 of the *Charter*. In addition, in most cases the financial costs of human rights litigation is a barrier to equity, since governments usually appeal first instance tribunal decisions granting new or expanded rights. Canadian human rights instruments thus have varying capacity to actually uphold the rights of citizens. Financial burdens are further amplified in British Columbia and Ontario, where governments have dispensed with the provision of investigative services to complainants, who must now go directly to the respective tribunals and from there, appeal to the courts, at their own cost. Table 13.1 summarizes the complaint process and the jurisdictional boundaries of these instruments.

As Table 13.1 confirms, the complaint process is arduous, and complainants usually bear the legal costs, which are substantial, unless litigation is funded by an interested organization, such as the Women's Legal Education and Action Fund (LEAF, 2010). LEAF is a national charitable organization that works toward ensuring the law guarantees substantive equality for all women in Canada. Its mandate is to ensure that the rights of women and

Table 13.1. Canadian Human Rights Instruments			
Canadian Human Rights Instruments	Process for Making a Complaint	Jurisdiction	Barriers to Access and Efficacy of Instrument
Charter of Rights & Freedoms (1982, 1985) Schedule B Constitution Act, 1982	No direct complaint mechanism. *Charter* arguments must be made at a tribunal, or at federal and provincial courts, and typically must be taken to the Supreme Court of Canada for final determination.	Federal Parliament and government of Canada. Legislature and government of each province and territory.	Right to health and redress for poverty and other forms of social inequity or exclusion would be difficult to argue as guaranteed by the *Charter* — they are not likely to be deemed analogous to the existing grounds under s. 15(1). s. 15(1) is subject to s. 1: "Rights and freedoms subject to 'reasonable limits prescribed by law as can be demonstrably justified in a free and democratic society.'" Require legal representation with prohibitive costs.

Table 13.1. Canadian Human Rights Instruments			
Canadian Human Rights Act R.S.C. 1985, c. H-6	Complaint to Canadian Human Rights Commission; Commission investigates and may send to Canadian Human Rights Tribunal; right of appeal to Federal Court and Supreme Court of Canada	Federally regulated organizations including employers, unions and service providers.	Right to health and redress for poverty and other forms of social inequity or exclusion not within scope of the Act. Potential legal costs for own lawyer as the Commission represents the public interest, not the complainant.
Provincial and Territorial Human Rights Legislation	Internal complaint process through the respective provincial or territorial commission. Commissions investigate complaints and represent the complainant at the tribunal and on appeals through the courts (with the exception of British Columbia and Ontario).	Public or private sector employers, service providers, organizations.	Right to health and redress for poverty and other forms of social inequity or exclusion not within scope of these statutes. Potential legal costs for own lawyer — commissions represent the public interest, not the complainant

girls, as guaranteed in the *Charter*, are upheld in our courts, human rights commissions and government agencies; and to take actions to reveal how factors such as race, class, Aboriginal status, sexual orientation, ability and religion compound discrimination against women. Since its inception in 1985, LEAF has intervened in over 150 cases and has helped establish landmark legal victories for women on a wide range of issues from violence against women, sexual assault, workplace inequities, socio-economic rights and reproductive freedoms (LEAF, 2010). LEAF intervened in the *Eldridge* case, discussed above, involving hearing impaired persons seeking medical care. LEAF also intervened in a case where it was ruled that a woman is entitled to share a couple's Canada Pension Plan credits if there is a separation or divorce (LEAF, 1990). This case was an important step in reducing older women's vulnerability to poverty. Programs such as LEAF are under persistent threat of decreased funding under current federal government cutbacks to agencies that advocate for discriminated persons and groups.

Further eroding citizen capacity to have their *Charter* rights upheld, in 2006, the federal government cancelled the Court Challenges Program — a national non-profit organization set up in 1994 to provide financial assistance for important court cases that advance language and equality rights guaranteed under Canada's Constitution.

> The Court Challenges Program, by providing modest contributions to the cost of important test cases dealing with language and equality rights, has made these constitutional rights accessible to Canadians. Without the Court Challenges Program, Canada's constitutional rights are real only for the wealthy. This is unfair. And it does not comply with the rule of law, which is a fundamental principle of our Constitution. (LEAF, 2004).

Another example of the erosion of human rights justiciability was the 1990s termination of the Equality Rights Program, which effectively extinguished access to funding for legal costs, including to such organization as LEAF and anti-poverty groups. A further burden for citizens in terms of the upholding of *Charter* rights and freedoms is the fact that citizens pay, through their taxes, government appeals for equitable remedies that may be ordered by tribunals and courts. The following example illustrates further barriers in achieving individual and group *Charter* rights.

Democratic Racism: An Example of Barriers to Human Rights Accountability

Ostensibly, Canadian citizens have strong human rights protection under the law, and human rights commissions have been set up in all provinces to ensure that these rights are upheld. However, even a cursory examination

Box 13.1 Case Example: Human Rights Codes and Commissions

The present model of human rights has been criticized for being a reactive model that comes into play only when a complaint is launched. Critics argue that commissions do not have a sufficiently broad mandate to combat discrimination effectively. A principal criticism is that a complaint-motivated system cannot effectively address a problem that is so wide-spread in society. The Canadian human-rights commissioner Maxwell Yalden reinforced the criticism of the complaint model: "I am convinced that one of the reasons our scheme of human-rights laws has become prey to bureaucratic delays and judicial haggling is that it so predominantly a complaint-driven model," which requires several conditions to be met: a victim must come forward; that person must be able to relate particular actions to one or more of the forbidden types of discrimination; and the treatment must be demonstrably discriminatory, not just unfair or different.

In resolving human-rights complaints, the present model allows for persuasion and conciliation where necessary and, alternatively, for punitive measures when such persuasion fails. Human-rights commissions are therefore under tremendous pressure to settle complaints. In attempting to reach conciliation, staff are often unaware of the impact of their behaviour on victims. In the hearings of a task force established to examine the procedures of the Ontario Human Rights Commission, delegations representing various community groups stated that the "process can be coercive and unfair. Claimants argued that sometimes they are specifically told that if they do not accept a settlement, which in their view is unjust, their case will be dismissed by the commission. Since they have no other choice, they feel forced to accept the settlement" (Ontario Human Rights Commission, 1992).

This complaint-driven approach is viewed as inadequate in addressing the complex, pervasive, and intractable forms of racism in Canadian society. A re-evaluation of the "effectiveness of a human rights system that is based on a model developed in the 1960's" (Mendes, 1997:2.v.) is clearly called for. Yalden concluded his analysis of human-rights commissions by noting that the human-rights system existing in most jurisdictions in Canada is not affording the victims of discrimination the recourse necessary to enforce their rights. In particular, cases of racial discrimination are proving to be too much for the present system to handle (Mendes, 1997).

Source: Henry, F., Tator, C., Mattis, W & Rees. T. (2000). The color of democracy: Racism in Canadian society. Toronto: Harcourt Canada. (p. 341–43)

of the processes and procedures involved in ensuring one's rights reveals critical drawbacks in human rights accountability. The case study in Box 13.1 details barriers in the justicability of these commissions. It illustrates democratic racism, where policies and laws designed within the principles of democracy in a democratic country, by democratically elected officials, often reinforce oppressions and perpetuate oppressive acts. As Henry et al. (2000) argue, human rights codes and commissions place the burden of responsibility on the individual rather than on the state. It is difficult to imagine what this burden might be like unless you have personal experience or have witnessed or assisted another person in navigating a complaints process. The complainant, and in many cases their families, must have a considerable reserve of mental and physical energy to withstand the close and sometimes damning scrutiny of counter-arguments. Inquiries or investigative processes can take months or years to come to a conclusion and can result in significant financial strain for the complainant and their family (McGibbon & Etowa, 2009).

As indicated in Table 13.1, in the provinces and territories, claims must be handled by a human rights commission, which investigates the claims and undertakes a process of potential settlement through conciliation and mediation. If this is not possible, the commission either dismisses the claim or sends it to hearings conducted by a human rights board of inquiry – a quasi-judicial tribunal which acts independently of the human rights commission. "If a claim goes to a board of inquiry, lawyers acting for the commission present the case and argue for the 'appropriate' remedy. Boards of inquiry make decisions to uphold or reject claims and can order redress, such as back pay and damages" (Henry, Tator, Mattis, & Rees, 2000, p. 343).

Democratic racism not only illustrates the significant barriers inherent in a complaints-based system for upholding individual human rights, it also provides a clear example of the limitations of human rights legal instruments and human rights commissions in supporting the rights of collectives of oppressed peoples.

Collective Accountability Exemplar:
A Human Rights-Based Health Report Card

Human rights-based report cards hold great promise for identifying adherence to collective rights and explicitly supporting policy change to decrease discrimination and oppression related to the right to health care and health protection. Monitoring a nation's progress on health outcomes is one way to hold governments accountable for their civic duty to citizens. The following sections briefly describe some important aspects of the development of a rights-based health report card (RBHRC) for Canadian jurisdictions (McGibbon, Etowa, & McPherson, 2008b). The goals of the RBHRC are to promote and support government accountability regarding achieving equity in Canadian health care access and ultimately to act as a catalyst for policy change in Canadian health and social policy related to health systems delivery. The RBHRC has the same goal as the U.S. civil rights report cards: the monitoring of progress toward equitable health care and health outcomes and the building of enduring trust in equitable treatment (Smith, 1998).

Health report cards are already available on a wide variety of indicators in Canada. For example, the Heart and Stroke Foundation (HSF) has produced a number of report cards regarding the cardiac status of Canadians. Its report on the gender gap in heart health recommended that the government conduct ongoing population surveillance of women's health outcomes and monitor and evaluate health services and community supports (HSF, 2007). The HSF noted that it is important to address socioeconomic determinants of women's heart diseases, such as poverty, geography, women's roles and control over their lives, and equality of access to services. Although there are a variety of health related report cards in Canada, we lack a comprehensive system to track adherence to the *Charter* areas of non-discrimination, including race, ethnicity and gender, to name a few.

In order to effectively track progress in these areas, it is imperative that government initiatives develop *equity specific* strategies for data collection and dissemination. For example, a gender lens is increasingly being used to assess policy intervention in Canada and globally. The distinct feature of the RBHRC is its dedicated and explicit goal of tracking the health effects of oppression. Human rights monitoring of health care access and health protection is in its very beginning in Canada. The First Nations Health Reporting Framework (FNHRF) is one of the first explicit strategies to monitor the health status of oppressed peoples in Canada. The goal of the FNHRF was to "develop a basic conceptual structure of First Nations specific health indicators that can be used to evaluate the success or failure of federal, provincial, and territorial governments in improving the health status of First Nations" (Assembly of First Nations, 2007: 4).

Much work has been done, particularly in the United States, to develop national strategies to measure a nation's progress in the area of health and health care access. McGibbon (2008) used two well-recognized and internationally respected templates for the initial development of the rights-based health report card: 1) civil rights monitoring and report cards (Smith, 2005a, 2005b, 1998) and 2) the equity gauge (Global Equity Gauge Alliance, 2003). In the U.S., Smith advocated for civil rights report cards, which focus specifically on the effects of discrimination on health outcomes of racialized peoples. This approach could be adapted for Canada to provide timely data to more directly address health inequities based in oppression. Smith's report card includes numerous health indicators, such as cardiovascular disease and cancer rates,

Table 13.2: A Rights-based Health Report Card for Canadian Jurisdictions		
Unit of Analysis	Data Source	Indicators by *Charter* Area of Non-Discrimination (Age, Race, Gender and Sexual Orientation)
Geographically Defined Population (by province, territory)	Canadian Institute of Health Information	1. total age adjusted death rate 2. cardiovascular death rate 3. infant death rate 4. children in families below LICO 5. suicide death rate by age
Geographically Defined Population (by province, territory, District Health Region)	Canadian Cancer Registry, National Pollution Release Inventory	1. lung cancer death rate 2. breast cancer death rate 3. prostate cancer death rate 4. colorectal cancer death rate 5. geographic incidence of environmental toxin related cancers: breast and prostate
Persons Admitted to Hospitals	MSI Provincial Administrative Databases	Sample Indicators (full list is comprehensive) *Mental Health Indicators* 1. % persons with suicidality as chief reason for admission (under 10; 10-19; 20-35; 36-50; 50-64; 65+) 2. % persons with depression as chief reason for admission (under 10; 10-19; 20-35; 36-50; 50-64; 65+) *Obstetric Indicators* 1. % low birthweight infants 3. % neonates with an APGAR 3 or less at 5 minutes, and a birthweight of <1500 grams *Oncology Indicators* 1. % survival of patients with primary cancer of the lung, colon/rectum, by stage & histology type 2. % referral for related tests critical to diagnosis, prognosis, and treatment *Cardiovascular Indicators* 1. % intra-hospital cardiovascular mortality (as a means of assessing multiple aspects of CABG-'bypass' care) 2. % extended postoperative stay (as a means of assessing multiple aspects of CABG).

Table 13.2: A Rights-based Health Report Card for Canadian Jurisdictions		
Persons Visiting Health Care Professionals the community	MSI Provincial Administrative Databases	1. % women for whom pre-natal care began in the first trimester 2. % children receiving all childhood immunization
Persons visiting Health Care Professionals in community	Canadian Community Health Survey (CCHC)	1. % 12 and over who visited a HCP in the last three years 3. % for whom last visit to doctor fully met their needs (Note: The CCHS focuses on doctors as the primary care practitioner)

as well as data from self reported national surveys. In the development of the Canadian RBHRC, we added more focus on mental health and a section designed to provide evidence of the geographic and demographic relationships among industrial pollutants and lung, breast, prostate and colorectal cancer rates. Table 13.2 builds on previous work (McGibbon, Etowa & McPherson, 2008b) as well as ongoing RBHRC grant proposal development. It includes corresponding units of analysis, Canadian data sources and indicators by *Charter* areas of non-discrimination. The full RBHRC includes over forty indicators. Table 13.2 includes sample indicators.

The initial development of the RBHRC must begin with nation-wide partnerships with key stakeholders in community and government and non-governmental organizations. One of the barriers to the creation of the RBHRC is the absence of health data coded for the *Charter* areas of non-discrimination in national data repositories such as Statistics Canada, the Canadian Institute for Health Information and the Canadian Cancer Registry. Some information is increasingly available, including social determinants of health data such as level of education for Aboriginal peoples by province. However, in area such as racism, key indicators, such as breast cancer incidence in women of colour versus referral rates for specialist intervention, are not yet consistently or comprehensively available in Canada. As Smith (1998: 78) points out, the monitoring of civil rights through the use of health monitoring report cards is a complex undertaking: "It is admittedly, a large, complex, and emotionally laden topic. In an area such as this, where there has been no rigorous empirical research, it may not be possible to do objective research. Indeed, it is hard enough just to have calm and open exchanges about the issues." A rights-based health report card serves the dual purposes of measuring and monitoring health outcomes across *Charter* areas of non-discrimination and of creating a proxy measurement of access to care for these equity-seeking groups. Access to care is much more difficult to quantify because it involves a synergy of individual stereotyping and discrimination with systemic discrimination against equity-seeking groups.

International Human Rights Law

Canada is a signatory to a number of international conventions, covenants and protocols that expressly address a wide range of human rights issues. Relevant documents include the United Nations Universal Declaration of Human Rights (1948), the International Covenant on Economic, Cultural and Social Rights (1966) and the Convention on the Elimination of all Forms of Discrimination against Women (1979). The latter convention obligates the state to uphold the right of rural women to "have access to adequate health care facilities, including information, counseling and services in family planning... to enjoy living conditions, particularly in relation to housing, sanitation, electricity and water supply, transport and communications" (United Nations, 1979). The Convention on the Rights of the Child (1989), Article 24, requires that states "recognize the right of the child to the enjoyment of the highest attainable standard of health and to facilities for the treatment of illness and rehabilitations of health... and strive to ensure that no child is deprived of his or her right of access to such health care services" (United Nations, 1989). Table 13.3 provides a complete list of relevant instruments.

On the face of these documents, access to equitable health care and health protection should be a given. Canadian Heritage is the federal government department with primary responsibility for oversight and reporting to the U.N. on the status of human rights in Canada. Its Human Rights Program website states: "U.N. conventions do not legislate rights, but recognize them and build upon them, principally by using moral suasion, education and public opinion." There are several potential processes for making a complaint, one of which requires that there be an "optional protocol" to the covenant or convention in question. Canada has signed optional protocols with respect to

Table 13.3 United Nations Human Rights Instruments
Universal Declaration of Human Rights (1948)
International Covenant on Civil and Political Rights (1966)
International Covenant on Economic, Social and Cultural Rights (1966)
International Convention on the Elimination of All Forms of Racial Discrimination (1966)
Convention on the Rights of the Child (1989)
Convention on the Elimination of Discrimination Against Women (1979)
Convention on the Rights of Persons with Disabilities (2006)

the International Covenant on Civil and Political Rights and the Convention on the Elimination of Discrimination Against Women.

Under these protocols Canadian citizens can make complaints to the Commission on Human Rights and the Commission on the Status of Women, if they have exhausted domestic remedies. The federal government is a participant, if it chooses to be, throughout the process. The commission will often entertain or seek submissions from interested third-party non-governmental organizations and agencies. If the commission decides that there has been a violation of the rights in question, it will ask Canada to indicate what steps it will take to address this violation. However, the findings of these commissions are not legally binding and Canada is not legally obligated to implement their recommendations. In summary, although U.N. human rights instruments are explicit in characterizing people's needs as rights, without legal enforceability, these instruments are largely ineffective, other than being useful for exploring Canada's shortfalls.

Economic Globalization and Human Rights

Human rights laws do not necessarily offer protection in the context of globalization because these laws were developed at a time when the state was the primary actor in international relations According to De Feyter (2005: 1), "The international human rights system was similarly state oriented. Domestic states carried human rights obligations *vis-à-vis* their citizens but not *vis-à-vis* anyone else." The human rights system thus relies on individuals being connected to a nation state with the capacity to protect its citizens.

De Feyter (2005) defines economic globalization as the breaking down of states' borders to allow the free flow of finance, trade, production and labour. He argues that human rights and social justice in the age of the market must be considered in light of three key areas. First, existing state obligations in the field of human rights must be rethought because state action is enhanced, or fettered, by the global market. In the case of water, for example, a state may jeopardize citizens' access to water by privatizing its water supply through agreements with a transnational water company, all the while being bound by human rights covenants and treaties to provide a safe supply of water.

Second, DeFeyter (2005: 3) argues that if human rights are to make a difference, "they should focus on empowering those who suffer the worst abuse. The experience of people alienated by the globalization process should inform the direction of the human rights project, rather than the extent to which dominant actors are willing to accommodate aspects of human rights that serve their interests." Chapter 11 describes some of the details of the civil society engagement that is crucial to a participatory approach to tackling inequities in the right to health.

Third, there must be a critical and systematic accounting for actors that are now central in the global context of human rights: multinational economic institutions and agreements (DeFeyter, 2005), including the General Agreement on Tarrifs and Trades (GATT),the World Trade Organization (WTO), the International Monetary Fund (IMF), the World Bank, and transnational companies, such as those that have an increasing control over global water supplies. For example, in 1993, the year of its inception, the World Bank adopted the Water Resources Management policy paper, which noted the unwillingness of poor countries to pay for their water services and stated that water should be treated as an economic commodity, with an emphasis on efficiency, financial discipline and full-cost recovery (Barlow, 2007).

The WTO continues to be a key actor in this age of the global market. Originally focused on agreements in the area of trade in goods, the WTO expanded the scope of globalization to include trade in services and the protection of intellectual property rights — Trade Related Aspects of Intellectual Property Rights (TRIPPS). A key problem with TRIPPS is its enhancement of transnational pharmaceutical companies, where maximizing profit, rather than increasing health and well-being, is the driving force. "The commercial nature of intellectual property protection means that patents provide incentives for research directed towards 'profitable' diseases, but not for research into diseases that predominately affect poor people" (DeFeyter 2005: 178). Furthermore, as discussed in Chapter 9, the overriding dominance of psychopharmaceutical intervention for oppression-related stress means that the industry continues to greatly profit from the maintenance of oppression.

Here, it is germane to note that in Canada, the fastest rising health expenditure is in pharmaceuticals (McGibbon, 2009). Drug therapies accounted for 9 percent of total health spending in 1975, and, by 2005, this figure nearly doubled, replacing payments to physicians as the second largest expenditure, behind hospitals (Health Canada, 2005). At the current rate, the $10 million spent on pharmaceuticals in 1996 will reach $85 billion by 2017, with one out of every four dollars spent on health care going to drugs (Morgan, 2006). This trend means that the transnational pharmaceutical industry has an influential political role in the shape and direction of Canada's vision of physical and mental health care. Since profit is the goal of the pharmaceutical industry, these statistics should be cause for concern and action, particularly since numerous scholars have linked oppression with over-medication or mis-medication of marginalized persons and groups. The following critical questions need to be publicly asked and debated: Through what political and policy based processes did the pharmaceutical industry gain such a massive share in Canadian health care expenditures? Who are the winners and who are the losers in the drive to make drugs a leading intervention in health care? These kinds of questions help to translate the complexity of economic globalization into a more practical, everyday realm.

Conclusions

There has been a great deal of work expended to enshrine human rights in numerous national and international legal instruments. Hence, there is a strong global will to set out the ways that justice may be served for citizens. The continued challenge is to translate these comprehensive human rights treaties and covenants into actual, on-the-ground strategies to ensure that the basic human necessities are available for a life with dignity, including access to health care and health protection. In the context of shifting global economic powers such as the WTO and the World Bank, it is increasingly difficult, not only to support a nation state's activities towards ensuring health as a human right, but also to even identify the locus of responsibility for human rights violations. Market-driven global interests continue to disrupt progress in attaining the human right to health. Critical analyses of economic globalization are urgently needed for development of a more advanced understanding of the human right to health and health protection. The concept of human rights involves complex local, national and global systems that are exceedingly difficult to disentangle. Ultimately, it is crucially important to continue to design ways to translate human rights instruments into measurable indicators of a state's capacity to provide equitable health care access as well as to protect the heath of its citizens within the context of economic globalization.

Select Bibliography

Abada, T., F. Hou and B. Ram. 2007. "Racially Mixed Neighborhoods, Perceived Neighborhood Social Cohesion, and Adolescent Health in Canada." *Social Science & Medicine* 65(10).

Abella, I., and H. Troper. 1983. *None Is Too Many: Canada and the Jews of Europe, 1933–1948.* Toronto: Lester and Orpen Dennys.

Adelman, R.D., M.G. Greene, R. Charon and E. Freidmann. 1990. "Issues in the Physician-Geriatric Patient Relationship." In H. Giles, N. Coupland, J.M. Wiemann (eds.), *Communication, Health and the Elderly.* New York: St. Martin's Press.

Agnew, V. 2002. *Gender, Migration and Citizenship Resources Project: Part II: A Literature Review and Bibliography on Health.* Toronto: Centre for Feminist Research, York University.

Ahmad, F., A. Shik, R. Vanza, A.M. Cheung, U. George and D.E. Stewart. 2004. "Voices of South Asian Women: Immigration and Mental Health." *Women & Health* 40(4).

Ahmed, A.T., S.A. Mohammed and D.R. Williams. 2007. "Racial Discrimination and Health: Pathways and Evidence." *Indian Journal of Medical Research* 126.

Alaimo, K., C.N. Olsen and E.A. Frongillo. 2002. "Family Food Insufficiency Is Positively Associated with Dysthymia and Suicide Symptoms in Adolescents." *American Society for Nutritional Sciences Journal of Nutrition* 132.

Albaek, E. 1995. "Between Knowledge and Power: Utilization of Social Science in Public Policy-Making." *Policy Sciences* 28(1).

Albrecht, D. 1998. "Community Health Centres in Canada." *Leadership in Health Services* 11(1).

Alcutias, H., L. Alcuitas-Imperial, C. Diocsan and J. Ordinario. 1997. *Trapped: "Holding on to the Knife's Edge": Economic Violence Against Filipino Migrant/ Immigrant Women.* Vancouver: Philippine Women's Centre of B.C.

Alesina, A., and E.L. Glaeser. 2004. *Fighting Poverty in the US and Europe: A World of Difference.* Toronto: Oxford University Press.

Ali, A., N. Massaquoi and M. Brown. 2003. "Racial Discrimination as a Health Risk for Female Youth: Implications for Policy and Health Care Delivery in Canada." *Directions: Research Reviews from the Canadian Race Relations Foundation* 1(2).

Alleyne, J., I. Papadopoulos and M. Tilki. 1994. "Anti-Racism within Transcultural Nurse Education." *British Journal of Nursing* 3(15).

Allison, K., E. Adlaf, A. Ialomiteanu and J. Rehm. 1999. "Predictors of Health Risk Behaviours among Young Adults: Analysis of the National Population Health Survey." *Canadian Journal of Public Health* 90(2).

Alzheimers Society of Canada. 2009. *Rising Tide: Impact of Dementia on Canadian Society.* Toronto: Alzheimers Society of Canada.

American Heart Association. 2001. *Heart and Stroke Statistical Update.* Retrieved on March 20, 2001 from <www.americanheart.org/statistics/stroke.html>.

American Psychiatric Association 2004. *Diagnostic and Statistical Manual of Mental Disorders: Text Revised*. Arlington, VA: American Psychiatric Association.

Amin, S. 1988. *Eurocentrism*. New York: Monthly Review Press.

Amnesty International and International Human Rights Network. 2005. *Our Rights, Our Future, Human Rights Based Approaches in Ireland: Principles, Policies and Practice*. <ihrnetwork.org/files/IHRNAI%20HRBA%20Ireland%20Sept05%20 FINAL.pdf>.

Anderson, J. 2000. "Gender, Race, Poverty, Health and Discourses of Health Reform in the Context of Globalization: A Post-Colonial Feminist Perspective in Policy Research." *Nursing Inquiry* 7(4).

Anderson, J., and S. Reimer-Kirkham. 1998. "Constructing Nation: The Gendering and Racializing of the Canada Health Care System." In Veronica Strong-Boag, Sherill Grace et al. (eds.), *Painting the Maple: Essays on Race, Gender, and the Construction of Canada*. Vancouver, BC: UBC Press.

Anderson, M.L., and P.H. Collins. 2007. *Race, Class, and Gender: An Anthology* (fifth ed.). Belmont, CA: Wadsworth Publishing.

Anderson W. 2002. *The Cultivation of Whiteness: Science, Health and Racial Destiny in Australia*. Melbourne, AU: Melbourne University Press.

Andrews v. Law Society of British Columbia. 1989. CanLII 2 (S.C.C.), p. 4. <canlii.org/ en/ca/scc/doc/1989/1989canlii2/1989canlii2.pdf>.

Angus, J., and P. Reeve. 2006. "Ageism: A Threat to 'Aging Well' in the 21st Century." *Journal of Applied Gerontology* 25(2).

Armstrong, H., and P. Armstrong. 2003. *Wasting Away: The Undermining of Canadian Health Care*. Toronto: Oxford University Press.

Armstrong, P. 2006. "Gender, Health and Care." In D. Raphael, T. Bryant and M. Rioux (eds.), *Staying Alive: Critical Perspectives on Health, Illness and Health Care*. Toronto: Canadian Scholars Press.

Arundel, K., and Associates. 2009. *How Are Canadians Really Doing: A Closer Look at Select Groups*. Toronto: Institute of Wellbeing.

Asquith, N. 2009. "Positive Ageing, Neoliberalism and Australian Sociology." *Journal of Sociology* 45(3).

Assembly of First Nations. 2007. *First Nations Regional Longitudinal Health Survey*. Ottawa.

Association of Ontario Health Centres. 2007. *Taking Action on the Social Determinants of Health*. Toronto: Association of Ontario Health Centres.

Atkinson, S. 2002. "Political Cultures, Health Systems and Health Policy." *Social Science and Medicine* 55.

Augoustinos, M., K. Tuffin and M. Rapley. 1999. "Genocide or a Failure to Gel? Racism, History and Nationalism in Australian Talk." *Discourse & Society* 10.

Australian Bureau of Statistics and Australian Institute of Health and Welfare. 2005. *The Health and Welfare of Australia's Aboriginal and Torres Strait Islander Peoples*. (ABS catno. 4704.0). Canberra, AU: Australian Government Printing Service.

Baltes, M.M., and L.L. Carstensen. 1996. "The Process of Successful Aging." *Ageing & Society* 16.

Bambra, C. 2009. "Welfare State Regimes and the Political Economy of Health." *Humanity and Society* 33.

___. 2007. "Going Beyond the Three Worlds of Welfare Capitalism: Regime Theory and Public Health Research." *Journal of Epidemiology and Community Health* 61(12).

Bambra, C., and T. Eikemo. 2008. "Welfare State Regimes, Unemployment and Health: A Comparative Study of the Relationship Between Unemployment and Self-Reported Health in 23 European Countries." *Journal of Epidemiology and Community Health* 63.

Bambra, C., D. Fox and A. Scott-Samuel. 2005. "Towards a Politics of Health." *Health Promotion International* 20(2).

Bannerji, H. 2004. "Immigrant Women: Labour in the North American Continent." In M. Bhattacharya (ed.), *Globalization*. New Delhi: Tulika Books.

Banting, K. 2005. "Canada: Nation-building in a Federal Welfare State." In Herbert Obinger, Stephan Leibfried and Francis G. Castles (eds.), *Federalism and the Welfare State: New World and European Experiences*. Cambridge: Cambridge University Press.

Barlow, M. 2007. *Blue Covenant: The Global Water Crisis and the Coming Battle for the Right to Water*. Toronto: McClelland and Stewart.

Bartky, S.L. 1990. *Femininity and Domination: Studies in the Phenomenology of Domination*. New York: Routledge.

Bassett, R., and J.E. Graham. 2007. "Memorabilities: Enduring Relationships, Memories and Abilities in Dementia." *Aging & Society* 27.

Battiste, M. 2000. *Reclaiming Indigenous Voice and Vision*. Vancouver: University of British Columbia Press.

Bauder, H. 2003. "'Brain Abuse,' or the Devaluation of Immigrant Labour in Canada." *Antipode* 35(4).

Beasley, R., M. Masoli, D. Fabian and S. Holt 2004. "The Global Burden of Asthma Report." *Allergy* 59(5).

Begley, S. 1996. "Three Is Not Enough: Surprising New Lessons from the Controversial Science of Race." *Newsweek 13*.

Belle, D., and J. Doucet. 2003. "Poverty, Inequality, and Discrimination as Sources of Depression among U.S. Women." *Psychology of Women Quarterly* 27(2).

Benach, J., Y. Yasui, C. Borrell, M. Sáez and M. Pasarin. 2001. "Material Deprivation and Leading Causes of Death by Gender: Evidence from a Nation-wide Small Area Study." *Journal of Epidemiology and Community Health* 55.

Bennett, M., and C. Blackstock. 2007. "Editorial." *First Peoples Child & Family Review* 3(3).

Benoit, C., D. Carroll and M. Chaudhry. 2003. "In Search of a Healing Place: Aboriginal Women in Vancouver's Downtown Eastside." *Social Science & Medicine* 56(4).

Benzeval, M., A. Dilnot, K. Judge and J. Taylor. 2001. "Income and Health over the Lifecourse: Evidence and Policy Implications." In H. Graham (ed.), *Understanding Health Inequalities*. Buckingham, UK: Open University Press.

Berg K., V, Bonham, J. Boyer, L. Brody, L. Brooks, F. Collins et al. 2005. "The Use of Racial, Ethnic, and Ancestral Categories in Human Genetics Research." *American Journal of Human Genetics* 77(4).

Bernard, W. 2002. "Including Black Women in Health and Social Policy Development: Winning over Addictions." In C. Amaratunga (ed.), *Race, Ethnicity and Women's Health*. Halifax, NS: Halcraft Printers.

Beyrer, C., and H.F. Pizer. 2007. *Public Health & Human Rights: Evidence-Based*

Approaches. Baltimore, MD: Johns Hopkins University Press.

Bhalla, R.K., M.A. Butters, J.T. Becker, P.R. Houck, B.E. Snitz, O.L. Lopez et al. 2009. "Patterns of Mild Cognitive Impairment after Treatment of Depression in the Elderly." *American Journal of Geriatric Psychiatry* 17(4).

Blaut, J.M. 1993. *The Colonizer's Model of the World: Geographical Diffusionism and Eurocentric History*. New York: Guildford Press.

Bobrow, D.B., and J.S. Dryzek 1987. *Policy by Design*. Pittsburgh: Pittsburg University Press.

Bond, C.J. 2005. "A Culture of Ill Health: Public Health or Aboriginality?" *Medical Journal of Australia* 183(1).

Bourgeault, I. 2006. "Sociological Perspectives on Health and Health Care." In D. Raphael, T. Bryant and M. Rioux (eds.), *Staying Alive: Critical Perspectives on Health, Illness, and Health Care*. Toronto: Canadian Scholars' Press, Inc.

Boyer, Y. 2003. *Aboriginal Health: A Constitutional Rights Analysis*. Native Law Centre and National Aboriginal Health Organization Discussion Paper Series on Aboriginal Health Paper No. 1.

Brady, D. 2003. "The Politics of Poverty: Left Political Institutions, the Welfare State, and Poverty." *Social Forces* 82.

Bramley, D., P. Hebert, L. Tuzzio and M. Chassin. 2005. "Disparities in Indigenous Health: A Cross-country Comparison between New Zealand and the United States." *American Journal of Public Health* 95.

Brancati, F.L., L. Kao, A.R. Folsom, R.L. Watson and M. Szklo. 2000. "Incident Type 2 Diabetes Mellitus in African American and White Adults: The Atherosclerosis Risk in Community Study." *Journal of the American Medical Association* 283(17).

Brandtstadter, J., and W. Greve. 1994. "'The Aging Self' Stabilizing and Protective Processes." *Developmental Review* 14.

Brave Heart, M.Y. 1999. "Gender Differences in the Historical Trauma Response Among the Lakota." *Journal of Health and Social Policy* 10(4).

Braveman, P., S. Egenter, C. Cubbin, and K. Marachi. 2001. "An Approach to Studying Social Disparities in Health and Health Care." *American Journal of Public Health* 91.

Braveman, P., and S. Gruskin. 2003. "Defining Equity in Health." *Journal of Epidemiology and Community Health* 57(4).

Breen, N., M. Wesley, R. Merril and K. Johnson. 2004. The Relationship of Socioeconomic Status and Access to Minimum Expected Therapy among Female Breast Cancer Patients in the Black-White Cancer Survival Study. *Ethnicity and Disease* 9.

Breggin, P.R. 2008. *Brain-Disabling Treatments in Psychiatry: Drugs, Electroshock and the Psychopharmaceutical Complex* (second ed.). New York: Springer Publishing Company.

Brodkin, K. 2000. *How Jews Became White folks*. New Brunswick, NJ: Rutgers University Press.

Brondolo, E. E.E. Love, M. Pencille, A. Schoenthaler and G. Ogedegbe. 2011. "Racism and Hypertension: A Review of the Empirical Evidence and Implications for Clinical Practice." *American Journal of Hypertension* 24 (May): 518–29.

Brondolo, E., N.B. ver Halen, M. Pencille, D. Beatty and R.J. Contrada. 2009. "Coping with Racism: A Selective Review of the Literature and a Theoretical and

Methodological Critique." *Journal of Behavioural Medicine* 32(1).

Brooks, S., and L. Miljan. 2003a. "Theories of Public Policy." In S. Brooks and L. Miljan (eds.), *Public Policy in Canada: An Introduction.* Toronto: Oxford University Press.

____. 2003b. *Public Policy in Canada: An Introduction.* Don Mills: Oxford University Press.

Brough, M.A. 1999. "A Lost Cause? Representations of Aboriginal and Torres Strait Islander Health in Australian Newspapers." *Australian Journal of Communication* 26(2).

Brown, D.R., V.M. Keith, J.S. Jackson and L. Gary. 2003. "(Dis)respected and (Dis) regarded: Experiences of Racism and Psychological Distress." In D.R. Brown and V.M. Keith (eds.), *In and Out of Our Right Minds: The Mental Health of African American Women.* New York: Columbia University Press.

Brunner, E. 1997. "Stress and the Biology of Inequality." *British Medical Journal* 314(7092).

Brunner, E., and M. Marmot. 2006. "Social Organization, Stress, and Health." In M. Marmot and R.G. Wilkinson (eds.), *Social Determinants of Health* (second ed.). Oxford: Oxford University Press.

Brunner, R.D. 1991. "The Policy Movement as a Policy Problem." *Policy Sciences* 24(1).

Bryant, T. 2009. *An Introduction to Health Policy.* Toronto: Canadian Scholars Press.

Bryant, T., S. Chisholm and C. Crowe. 2002. *Housing as a Determinant of Health.* The Social Determinants of Health Across the Life-Span Conference, Toronto.

Bryant, T., D. Raphael, T. Schrecker and R. Labonte. 2009. Canada: A land of Missed Opportunity for Addressing the Social Determinants of Health. Health Policy (2010), doi:10.1016/j.healthpol.2010.08.022. <http://www.hpclearinghouse.ca/pdf/missed%20opportunity%20sdoh.pdf>.

Buckley, N.J., F.T. Denton, A.L. Robb and B.G. Spencer. 2004. "Healthy Aging at Older Ages: Are Income and Education Important?" *Canadian Journal on Aging Supplement.*

Butler, J. 2001. "Giving an Account of Oneself." *Diacritics* 31.

____. 1990. *Gender Trouble: Feminism and the Subversion of Identity.* New York: Routledge.

Butler-Jones, D. 2008. *Report on the State of Public Health in Canada 2008.* Ottawa: Public Health Agency of Canada.

Byl, Y. 2009. *Entrenching Exploitation: Second Report of the AFL Temporary Foreign Worker Advocate.* Edmonton: Alberta Federation of Labour. <http://www.afl.org/index.php/Reports/entrenching-exploitation-second-rept-of-afl-temporary-foreign-worker-advocate.html>

Byrne, D. 1999. *Social Exclusion.* Buckingham, U.K.: Open University Press.

Calasanti, T. 2007. "Bodacious Berry, Potency, Wood and the Aging Monster: Gender and Age Relations in Anti-Aging Ads." *Social Forces* 86, 1 (September).

Calasanti, T., K.F. Slevin and N. King. 2006. "Ageism and Feminism: From 'et cetera' to Center." *National Women's Studies Association Journal* 18, 1 (Spring).

Calliste, A., and G.S. Dei. 2000. *Anti-Racist Feminism: Critical Race and Gender Studies.* Halifax, NS: Fernwood Publishing.

Campaign 2000. 2010. "2010 Report Card on Child and Family Poverty in Canada, 1989–2010." <http://www.campaign2000.ca/reportCards/national/2010Englis hC2000NationalReportCard.pdf>.

____. 2009. "2009 Report Card on Child and Family Poverty in Canada, 1989–2009." <http://www.campaign2000.ca/reportCards/national/2009EnglishC2000Natio nalReportCard.pdf>.

____. 2008. "2008 Report Card on Child and Family Poverty in Canada, 1989–2008." <http://www.campaign2000.ca/reportCards/national/2008EngNationalRepor tCard.pdf>.

Canadian Public Health Association. 2008. *Response of the Canadian Public Health Association to the Report of the World Health Organization's Commission on the Social Determinants of Health*. Ottawa: Canadian Public Health Association.

Caplan, P. 2004. *They Say You're Crazy: How the World's Most Powerful Psychiatrists Decide Who's Normal*. Reading, MA: Perseus Books.

Carstensen, L.L., and A.M. Freund. 1994. "Commentary: The Resiliency of the Aging Self." *Developmental Review* 14.

Cassidy, T. 1999. *Stress, Cognition, and Health*. New York: Routledge.

CCJA (Canadian Criminal Justice Association). 2000. "Aboriginal Peoples and the Criminal Justice system." May 15. *Bulletin of the CCJA*. Ottawa.

CCSD (Canadian Council on Social Development). 2009. "Protecting Canadians at Greatest Risk: Economic Recession and Poverty Reduction." Submission to federal pre-budget consultation. <ccsd.ca/ccsd-submission-pre-budget-consul.pdf>.

Centers for Disease Control and Prevention (CDCP). 2011. *Health Disparities and Inequality Report*. Atlanta: CDCP, 60 (Suppl).

Chan, M. 2009. "Steadfast in the Midst of Perils." Keynote address, Dr. Margaret Chan, Director-General of WHO, 12th World Congress on Public Health. Istanbul, Turkey. April 27. <who.int/dg/speeches/2009/steadfast_midst_perils_20090428/ en/index.html>.

Chernomas, R., and Hudson, I. 2009. "Social Murder: The Long-Term Effects of Conservative Economic Policy." *International Journal of Health Services* 39(1).

Chesterman, J., and B. Galligan. 1998. *Citizens Without Rights*. Cambridge: Cambridge University Press.

Choi, B.C.K., and F. Shi. 2001. "Risk Factors for Diabetes Mellitus by Age and Sex: Results of the National Population Health Survey." *Diabetologia* 44(10).

Choiniere, R., A. Lafontaine and A. Edwards. 2000. "Distribution of Cardiovascular Disease Risk Factors by Socioeconomic Status among Canadian Adults." *Canadian Medical Association Journal* 162.

Chronic Disease Alliance of Ontario. 2008. *Primer to Action: Social Determinants of Health*. Toronto: Chronic Disease Alliance of Ontario.

Chui, T. 2003. *Longitudinal Survey of Immigrants to Canada: Process, Progress and Prospects*. Ottawa: Statistics Canada.

CIC (Citizenship and Immigration Canada). 2009. *Facts and Figures: Immigration Overview Permanent and Temporary Residents 2008*. Ottawa: CIC. Minister of Public Works and Government Services Canada.

____. 2005. "Annual Report to Parliament on Immigration, 2005: Section 6, Gender-Based Analysis of the Impact of the Immigration and Refugee Protection Act." <cic.gc.ca/English/resources/publications/annual-report2005/section6.asp>.

CIHI (Canadian Institute for Health Information). 2008. *Reducing Gaps in Health: A Focus on Socio-Economic Status in Urban Canada*. Ottawa: Canadian Institutes for Health Research.

___. 2006. *Improving the Health of Canadians: An Introduction to Health in Urban Places*. Ottawa: CIHI. <http://secure.cihi.ca/cihiweb/products/PH_Full_Report_English.pdf>.

___. 2004. *Canadian Population Health Initiative*. Ottawa.

CIHR (Canadian Institutes for Health Research). 2009. *Funding Opportunities*. Ottawa:.

___. 2005. *Pathways and Gateways from Research to Policy: Focus on the Determinants of Immigrant Health*. <cihr-irsc.gc.ca/e/36695.html>.

Clark, M. 1972. "Cultural Values and Dependency in Later Life." In D.O. Cowgill and L.D. Holmes (eds.), *Aging and Modernization*. Norwalk, CT: Appleton-Century-Crofts.

Clarke, L.H., and M. Griffin. 2008. "Failing Bodies: Body Language and Multiple Conditions in Later Life." *Qualitative Health Research* 18(8).

Cloutterbuck, J., and D. Feeney Mahoney. 2003. "African American Dementia Caregivers: The Duality of Respect." *Dementia* 2, 221.

Coburn, D. 2006. "Health and Health Care: A Political Economy Perspective." In D. Raphael, T. Bryant and M. Rioux (eds.), *Staying Alive: Critical Perspectives on Health, Illness, and Health Care*. Toronto: Canadian Scholars Press.

___. 2003. "Income Inequality, Social Cohesion, and the Health Status of Populations: The Role of Neoliberalism." In R. Hofrichter (ed.), *Health and Social Justice: Politics, Ideology and Inequity in the Distribution of Disease*. San Francisco: Jossey-Bass.

Cochran, B., A.J. Stewart, J.A. Ginzler and A.M. Cauce. 2002. "Challenges Faced by Homeless Sexual Minorities: Comparison of Gay, Lesbian, Bisexual, and Transgender Homeless Adolescents with Their Heterosexual Counterparts." *American Journal of Public Health* 92(5).

Cohen, A. 1999. *The Mental Health of Indigenous Peoples: An International Overview*. Geneva: Nations for Mental Health, Department of Mental Health, World Health Organization.

Cohen, M.D., J.G. March and J.P. Olsen. 1972. "A Garbage Can Model of Organizational Choice." *Administrative Science Quarterly* 17(1).

Coker, E. 2004. "'Traveling Pains': Embodied Metaphors of Suffering Among Southern Sudanese Refugees in Cairo." *Culture, Medicine and Psychiatry* 28.

Coleman, W. 1982. *Death Is a Social Disease: Public Health and Political Economy in Early Industrial France*. Madison: University of Wisconsin Press.

Collins, P.H. 1990. *Black Feminist Thought: Knowledge, Consciousness, and the Politics of Empowerment*. Boston: Unwin Hyman.

Collins, P., J. Abelson and J. Eyles. 2007. "Knowledge into Action?: Understanding Ideological Barriers to Addressing Health Inequalities at the Local Level." *Health Policy* 80(1): 158–71.

Conference Board of Canada. 2008. *Healthy People, Healthy Performance, Healthy Profits: The Case for Business Action on the Socio-Economic Determinants of Health*. Ottawa: Conference Board of Canada.

___. 2006. *Performance and Potential: The World and Canada*. Ottawa: Conference Board of Canada.

___. 2003. *Defining the Canadian Advantage*. Ottawa: Conference Board of Canada.

Connett, M. 2003. "The Phosphate Fertilizer Industry: An Environmental Overview." Fluoride Action Network. <fluoridealert.org/phosphate/overview.htm#2>.

Conrad, P. 2005. "The Shifting Engines of Medicalization." *Journal of Health and Social Behaviour* 26.

Convention on the Elimination of All Forms of Discrimination Against Women. 1979. <un.org/womenwatch/daw/cedaw/>.

Cooper, R., J.S. Kaufman and R. Ward. 2003. "Race and Genomics." *New England Journal of Medicine* 348(12).

Cooper, G.S., Z. Yuan, A. Chak, and A. Rimm. 2000. "Patterns of Endoscopic Follow-Up after Surgery for Nonmetastatic Colorectal Cancer." *Gastrointestinal Endoscopy* 52(1).

Cooper, R., and C.N. Rotimi. 1997. "Hypertension in Blacks." *American Journal of Hypertension* 10.

Cowlishaw, G. 1997. "Where Is Racism?" In G. Cowlishaw and B. Morris (eds.), *Race Matters: Indigenous Australians and 'Our' Society*. Canberra, AU: Aboriginal Studies Press.

Coyte, P., and P. McKeever. 2001. "Home Care in Canada: Passing the Buck." *Canadian Journal of Nursing Research* 33(2).

CPHI (Canadian Population Health Initiative). 2004a. *Improving the Health of Canadians*. Ottawa: CPHI

___. 2004b. *Select Highlights on Public Views of the Determinants of Health*. Ottawa: CPHI.

___. 2002. *Canadian Population Health Initiative Brief to the Commission on the Future of Health Care in Canada*. <secure.cihi.ca/cihiweb/en/downloads/cphi_policy_romanowbrief_e.pdf>.

CRIAW (Canadian Research Institute for the Advancement of Women). 2006. *Intersectional Feminist Frameworks: A Primer*. Ottawa.

CSDH (Commission on the Social Determinants of Health). 2008. *Closing the Gap in a Generation: Health Equity Through Action on the Social Determinants Of Health*. Geneva: World Health Organization.

Cunneen C. 2001. "The Criminalisation of Indigenous People." In C. Cunneen (ed.), *Conflict, Politics and Crime: Aboriginal Communities and the Police*. Crows Nest, NSW: Allen and Unwin.

Cunningham, J., and J.R. Condon. 1996. "Premature Mortality in Aboriginal Adults in the Northern Territory, 1979–1991." *Medical Journal of Australia* 165.

Curry-Stevens, A. 2001. *When Markets Fail People: Exploring the Widening Gap Between Rich and Poor in Canada*. Toronto, ON: Canadian Social Justice Foundation for Research and Education.

Dahlgren G., and M. Whitehead. 1992. *Policies and Strategies to Promote Equity in Health*. Copenhagen: World Health Organization.

Danso, R. 2001. "From 'There' to 'Here': An Investigation of the Initial Settlement Experiences of Ethiopian and Somali Refugees in Toronto." *Geo-Journal* 55.

Davey Smith, G. (ed.). 2003. *Inequalities in Health: Life Course Perspectives*. Bristol UK: Policy Press.

Davis, D. 1997. "Blood and Nerves Revisited: Menopause and Privatization of the Body in a Newfoundland Postindustrial Fishery." *Medical Anthropology Quarterly* 11(1).

De Feyter, K. 2005. *Human Rights: Social Justice in the Age of the Market*. Halifax, NS: Fernwood Publishing.

Diamanti-Kandarakis, E., J-P. Bourguinon, L.C. Giudice, R. Hauser, G.S. Prins, A.M, Soto et al. 2009. "Endocrine-Disrupting Chemicals: An Endocrine Society Statement." *EndocrineReviews* 30(4). <http://www.endo-society.org/journals/scientificstatements/upload/edc_scientific_statement.pdf>.

Dillaway, H.E., and M. Byrnes. 2009. "Reconsidering Successful Aging: A Call for Renewed and Expanded Academic Critiques and Conceptualisations." *Journal of Applied Gerontology* 28.

Din-Dzietham, R., W.N. Nembhard, R. Collins, and S.K. Davis. 2004. "Perceived Stress Following Race-Based Discrimination at Work Is Associated with Hypertension in African-Americans. The Metro Atlanta Heart Disease Study, 1999–2001." *Social Science & Medicine* 58 (3).

Dodson, M. 1994. "The Wentworth Lecture: The End in the Beginning: Re(de)finding Aboriginality." *Australian Aboriginal Studies* 1.

Douglas Scott, S., A. Pringle and C. Lumsdaine. 2004. *Sexual Exclusion — Homophobia and Health Inequalities: A Review of Health Inequalities and Social Exclusion Experienced by Lesbian, Gay and Bisexual People.* UK Gay Men's Health Network. <http://www.spectrum-lgbt.org/downloads/health/gmhn_report.pdf>.

Doyal, L., and I. Pennell. 1979. *The Political Economy of Health.* London: Pluto Press.

Dressler, W. 2000. "Indigenous Societies." In E. Fink (ed.), *Encyclopedia of Stress.* San Diego: Academic Press.

____. 1991. *Stress and Adaptation in the Context of Culture: Depression in a Southern Black Community.* Albany: SUNY Press.

Drevdahl, D.J., M.K. Canales and K.S. Dorcy. 2008. "Of Goldfish Tanks and Moonlight Tricks: Can Cultural Competence Ameliorate Health Disparities?" *Advances in Nursing Science* 51(1).

Dugger, W.M. 1998. "Against Inequality." *Journal of Economic Issues* 32.

Duncan, C., and W. Loretto. 2004. "Never the Right Age? Gender and Age-Based Discrimination in Employment." *Gender, Work & Organization* 11(1).

Dunn, J., and I. Dyck. 2000. "Social Determinants of Health in Canada's Immigrant Population: Results from the National Population Health Survey." *Social Science and Medicine* 51(11).

____. 1998. *Social Determinants of Health in Canada's Immigrant Population: Results from the National Population Health Survey.* #98-20. Vancouver: Metropolis Project.

Duran, B., and E. Duran. 1995. *Native American Post-Colonial Psychology.* Albany, NY: State University of New York Press.

Durie, M. 1998. *Whaiora Maori Health Development* (second ed.). Auckland, NZ: Oxford University Press.

Dye, T.R. 1972. *Understanding Public Policy.* Englewood Cliffs, NJ: Prentice-Hall.

Dyer, S., and D. Woynillowicz. 2008. *Oil Sands Reclamation: Fact or Fiction?* Drayton Valley, AB: Pembina Institute.

Earle, C., L. Venditti, P. Neuman, R. Gelber, M. Weinstein, A. Potosky et al. 2000. "Who Gets Chemotherapy for Metastatic Lung Cancer?" *Chest* 117.

Eckersley, R. 1995. "Environmental Security Dilemmas: Review Article." *Environmental Politics* 5(1).

Eikemo, T.A., and C. Bambra. 2008. "The Welfare State: A Glossary for Public Health." *Journal of Epidemiology and Community Health* 62(1).

Eldridge v. British Columbia. 1997. Attorney General, 1997, CanLII 327 (S.C.C.). <canlii. org/en/ca/scc/doc/1997/1997canlii327/1997canlii327.pdf>.

Ellison, G.T.H. and I.R. Jones. 2002. "Social Identities and the 'New Genetics': Scientific and Social Consequences." *Critical Public Health* 12(3).

Enang [Etowa], J.E. 1999. "Childbirth Experiences of African Nova Scotian Women." Master of Nursing thesis, Dalhousie University, Halifax, NS.

____. 2002. "Black Women's Health: Health Research Relevant to Black Nova Scotians." In C. Amaratunga (ed.), *Race, Ethnicity and Women's Health*. Halifax, NS: Halcraft Printers.

Engels, F. 2009 [1845]. *The Condition of the Working Class in England*. New York: Penguin Classics.

Esping-Andersen, G. (ed.) 2002. *Why We Need a New Welfare State*. Oxford UK: Oxford University Press.

____. 1999. *Social Foundations of Post-Industrial Economies*. New York: Oxford University Press.

____. 1990. *The Three Worlds of Welfare Capitalism*. Princeton: Princeton University Press.

____. 1985. *Politics Against Markets: The Social Democratic Road to Power*. Princeton: Princeton University Press.

Essed, P. 1991. *Understanding Everyday Racism: An Interdisciplinary Theory*. Newbury Park, CA: Sage Publications.

Etowa, J. 2005. *Fostering Diversity in the Nursing Workforce: The Worklife Experiences of African Canadian Nurses*. International Council of Nurses (ICN) 23rd Quadrennial Congress. Taipei, Taiwan.

Etowa, J., B. Keddy, J. Egbeyemi and F. Eghan. 2007. "Depression: The 'Invisible Grey Fog': Influencing the Mental Health of African Canadian Women." *International Journal of Mental Health Nursing* 16.

Etowa, J., J. Weins, W.T. Bernard and B. Clow. 2007. "Determinants of Black Women's Health in Rural and Remote Communities." *Canadian Journal of Nursing Research* 39(3).

Evans, G., and K. English. 2002. "The Environment of Poverty: Multiple Stressor Exposure, Psychophysiological Stress, and Socioemotional Adjustment." *Child Development* 73(4).

Evans, G., and P. Kim. 2007. "Childhood Poverty and Health: Cumulative Risk Exposure and Stress Deregulation." *Psychological Science* 18(11).

Evans, G., and M. Schamberg. 2009. "Childhood Poverty, Chronic Stress, and Adult Working Memory." *Proceedings of the National Association of the Academy of Sciences* 106(16).

Eyles, J., M. Brimacombe, P. Chaulk, G. Stoddart, T. Pranger and O. Moase. 2001. "What Determines Health? To Where Should We Shift Resources? Attitudes Towards the Determinants of Health Among Multiple Stakeholder Groups in Prince Edward Island, Canada." *Social Science & Medicine* 53(12).

FAIA (Feminist Alliance for International Action). 2008. *Women's Inequality in Canada*. Submission of the Canadian FAIA to the United Nations Committee on the Elimination of Discrimination Against Women on the Occasion of the Committee's Review of Canada's 6th and 7th Reports.

Fanon F. 1963. *The Wretched of the Rarth*. New York: Grove Press.

Farmer, P. 2003. *Pathologies of Power: Health, Human Rights, and the New War on the Poor.* California Series in Public Anthropology, 4. Los Angeles, CA: University of California Press.

Featherstone, M., and M. Hepworth. 1995. "Images of Positive Ageing: A Case Study of Retirement Choice Magazine." In M. Featherston and A. Wernick (eds.), *Images of Aging: Cultural Representation of Later Life.* London: Routledge.

Featherstone, M., M. Hepworth and B.S. Turner (eds.). 1991. *The Body: Social Process and Cultural Theory.* London: Sage.

Fernando, S. 2003. *Cultural Diversity, Mental Health and Psychiatry: The Struggle Against Racism.* New York: Brunner-Routledge.

Ferraro, K.F., and T.P. Shippee. 2009. "Aging and Cumulative Inequality: How Does Inequality Get Under the Skin?" *The Gerontologist* 49(3).

Finkelstein, M. 2008. "The Prevalence of Diabetes Among Overweight and Obese Individuals is Higher in Poorer than in Richer Neighbourhoods." *Canadian Journal of Diabete* 32(3).

Fish, J. 2007. "Getting Equal: The Implications of New Regulations to Prohibit Sexual Orientation Discrimination for Health and Social Care." *Diversity in Health and Social Care* 4(3).

Fisher, B.J., and D.K. Specht. 1999. "Successful Aging and Creativity in Later Life." *Journal of Aging Studies* 13.

Fitzpatrick, T.R. 2009. "The Quality of Dyadic Relationships, Leisure Activities and Health Among Older Women." *Health Care for Women International* 30(12).

Fletcher, R.H., and S.W. Fletcher. 2005. *Epidemiology: The Essentials* (fourth ed.). New York: Lippincott, Williams and Wilkins.

Foucault, M. 1980. *Power/Knowledge: Selected Interviews and Other Writings, 1972–1977.* New York: Pantheon.

____. 1972. *The Archeology of Knowledge* (A.M. Sheridan-Smith, trans). London: Tavistock.

Franklin, D.C. 2002. "Racism Related Stress, Racial Identity, and Psychological Health for Blacks in America." Unpublished Doctoral dissertation, Columbia University.

Frankovits, A. 2006. *The Human Rights Based Approach and the United Nations System.* UNESCO Strategy on Human Rights: Social and Human Sciences Sector. France: UNESCO. <http://unesdoc.unesco.org/images/0014/001469/146999e.pdf>.

Fremstad, S. 2009. *Half in Ten: Why Taking Disability into Account is Essential to Reducing Income Poverty and Expanding Economic Inclusion.* Washington, DC: Center for Economic and Policy Research.

Fukuyama, F. 1996. *Trust: The Social Virtues and the Creation of Prosperity.* London: Penguin Books.

Galabuzi, G. 2006. *Canada's Economic Apartheid: The Social Exclusion of Racialized Groups in the New Century.* Toronto: Canadian Scholars Press.

____. 2004a. "Social Exclusion." In D. Raphael (ed.), *Social Determinants of Health: Canadian Perspectives.* Toronto: Canadian Scholars Press.

____. 2004b. "Racializing the Division of Labour: Neo-liberal Restructuring and the Economic Segregation of Canada's Racialized Groups." In J. Stanford and L. Vosko (eds.), *Challenging the Market: The Struggle to Regulate Work and Income.* Montreal/Kingston: McGill/Queens University Press.

____. 2001. *Canada's Creeping Economic Apartheid: The Economic Segregation and*

Social Marginalizaiton of Racialized Groups. <socialjustice.org/pubs/pdfs/economic_apartheid.pdf>.

Galvao, J. 2005. "Brazil and Access to HIV/AIDS Drugs: A Question of Human Rights and Public Health." *American Journal of Public Health* 95(7).

Gamble, A. 1988. *The Free Economy and the Strong State: The Politics of Thatcherism.* London: MacMillan.

Gardiner-Garden, J. 2003. *Defining Aboriginality in Australia.* Current Issues Brief No. 10 2002-03. Canberra, AU: Department of the Parliamentary Library.

Gardner, S.M. 2008. "Cure for Cancer? An Environmental Answer." Northeastern Nova Scotia Regional Science Fair, Port Hawkesbury, NS, Canada.

Gartner, R., and S. Thompson. 2004. "Trends in Homicide in Toronto." Paper presented at the University of Toronto Centre of Criminology Research Colloquium on Community Safety: From Enforcement and Prevention to Civic Engagement, Toronto, June 25.

Gary, F.A. 2005. "Stigma: Barrier to Mental Health Care among Ethnic Minorities." *Issues in Mental Health Nursing* 26.

Gasher, M. 2007. "Spreading the News: Social Determinants of Health Reportage in Canadian Daily Newspapers." *Canadian Journal of Communication* 32(3).

Gauri, V. 2003. *Social Rights and Economic Claims to Health Care and Education in Developing Countries.* World Bank Policy Research Working Paper 3006. Washington, DC: World Bank.

Gill, S.R. 1993. "Neoliberalism and the Shift towards a US-Centered Transnational Hegemony." In H. Overbeek (ed.), *Restructuring Hegemony in the Global Political Economy.* London: Routledge.

Gilmour, H. 2008. *Depression and Risk of Heart Disease.* Statistics Canada Catalogue no. 82-003-X. Ottawa.

Gilmore, J. 2004. *Health of Canadians Living in Census Metropolitan Areas.* Ottawa: Ministry of Industry.

Glaze, W.D., K.N. Anderson and L.E. Anderson (eds.). 1994. *Mosby's Medical, Nursing and Allied Health Dictionary.* St. Louis, MO: Mosby, Inc.

Glazier, R.H. and G. Booth. 2007. *Neighbourhood Environments and Resources for Healthy Living—A Focus on Diabetes in Toronto.* Toronto: Institute for Clinical Evaluative Sciences.

Global Equity Alliance. 2003. *The Equity Gauge: Concepts, Principles, and Guidelines.* Durban: Global Equity Alliance and Health Systems Trust.

Goddard, A.W., S.G. Ball, J. Martinez, C.R. Yang, J.M. Russell and A.Shekhar. 2010. "Current Perspectives of the Roles of the Central Norepinephrine System in Anxiety and Depression." *Depression and Anxiety* 27(4).

Goffman, E. 1961. *Asylums: Essays on the Social Situation of Mental Patients and Other Inmates.* New York: Anchor Books.

Gold, J., and M. Desmeules. 2004. "National Symposium on Immigrant Health in Canada." *Canadian Journal of Public Health* 95(3).

Goldstein, R.B., M. Olfson, P.J. Wickramaratne and S.I. Wolk. 2006. "Use of Outpatient Mental Health Services by Depressed and Anxious Children as They Grow Up." *Psychiatric Services* 57.

Goodstone, A., C. Quayle and P. Ranald. 2001. *Discrimination... Have You Got All Day? Indigenous Women, Discrimination and Complaints Processes in NSW.*

Sydney: Public Interest Advocacy Centre and Wirringa Baiya Aboriginal Women's Legal Centre.

Gorman S. 2004. "Moorditj Magic: The Story of Jim and Phillip Krakouer." Unpublished Doctoral dissertation. Perth: Edith Cowan University.

Government of Canada. 2006. *The Human Face of Mental Health and Illness in Canada, 2006.* Ottawa: Public Health Agency of Canada.

___. 1984. *Canada Health Act.* Ottawa, April 1: Parliament of Canada.

___. 1982a. *The Canada Charter of Rights and Freedoms.* Ottawa.

___. 1982b. *Constitution Act Part One: Canadian Charter of Rights and Freedoms,* Ottawa, March 29: Parliament of Canada.

Grabb, E. 2007. *Theories of Social Inequality* (fifth ed.). Toronto: Harcourt Canada.

Graham, H. 2004. "Social Determinants and Their Unequal Distribution: Clarifying Policy Understandings." *Milbank Quarterly* 82(1).

Green, A., D. Carney, D. Pallin, L. Ngo, C. Raymond, L. Iezzoni et al. 2007. "Implicit Bias Among Physicians and its Prediction of Thrombolysis Decisions for Black and White Patients." *Journal of General Internal Medicine* 22(9).

Green, A., and D. Green. 2004. "The Goals of Canada's Immigration Policy: A Historical Perspective." *Canadian Journal of Urban Research* 13(1).

Green, C.R., K.O. Anderson, T.A. Baker, L.C. Campbell, S. Decker, R. Fillingim et al. 2003. "The Unequal Burden of Pain: Confronting Racial and Ethnic Disparities in Pain." *Pain Medicine* 4(3).

Grieshaber-Otto, J., and S. Sinclair. 2004. *Bad Medicine: Trade Treaties, Privatization and Health Care Reform in Canada.* Ottawa: Canadian Centre for Policy Alternatives.

Grosfugel, R. 2004. "Race and Ethnicity or Racialized Ethnicities? Identities within Global Coloniality." *Ethnicities* 4(3).

Grove, N.J., and A.B. Zwi. 2006. "Our Health and Theirs: Forced Migration, Othering, and Public Health." *Social Science & Medicine* 62(8).

Gruskin, S., E.J. Mills and D. Tarantala. 2007. "Health and Human Rights I: History, Principles, and Practice of Health and Human Rights." *Lancet* 370.

Guba, E. (ed.). 1990. *The Paradigm Dialog.* Newbury Park CA: Sage.

Guehlstorf, N., and L.K. Hallstrom. 2005. "The Role of Culture in Risk Regulations: A Comparative Case Study of Genetically Modified Corn in the United States of America and the European Union." *Environmental Science and Policy* 8(4).

Gullette, M.M. 2004. *Aged by Culture.* Chicago: University of Chicago Press.

Gump, J.P. 2010. "Reality Matters: The Shadow of Trauma on African American Subjectivity." *Psychoanalytic Psychology* 27(1).

Haan, M. 2008. "The Place of Place: Location and Immigrant Economic Well-Being in Canada." *Population Research and Policy Review* 27.

Halli, S., and A. Kazemipur. 2001. "The Changing Colour of Poverty in Canada." *Canadian Review of Sociology and Anthropology* 38(2).

Ham, C., and M. Hill. 1984. *The Policy Process in the Modern Capitalist State.* Brighton, UK: Wheatsheaf Books.

Hankivsky, O., and A. Christoffersen. 2008. Intersectionality and the Determinants of Health: A Canadian Perspective. *Critical Public Health* 18(3).

Hankivsky, O., and R. Cormier. 2010. "Intersectionality and Public Policy: Some Lessons from Existing Models." *Political Research Quarterly* 63(2).

Hankivsky, O., R. Cormier and D. de Merich. 2009. *Intersectionality: Moving Women's Health Research and Policy Forward*. Vancouver: Women's Health Research Network.

Harrell, J.P., S. Hall and J. Taliaferro. 2003. "Physiological Responses to Racism and Discrimination: An Assessment of the Evidence." *American Journal of Public Health* 93(2).

Harry, R. 2008. "The British Columbia Restorative Health Project." Victoria: British Columbia Aboriginal Network on Disability Society. <bcands.bc.ca/G.%20 Kiesman/BC%20Aboriginal%20Restorative%20Health%20Project%20 Summary.pdf>.

Hatch, C., and M. Price. 2008. *Canada's Toxic Tar Sands: The Most Destructive Project on Earth*. Toronto: Environmental Defense.

Havemann P. 1999 *Indigenous Peoples' Rights in Australia, Canada and New Zealand*. Auckland: Oxford University Press.

Havighurst, R.J. 1961. "Successful Aging." *Gerontologist* 1: 8–13.

Hayes, M., I. Ross, M. Gasherc, D. Gutstein, J. Dunn and R. Hackett. 2007. "Telling Stories: News Media, Health Literacy and Public Policy in Canada." *Social Science and Medicine* 54.

Health Canada. 2005. *Canada's Health Care System*. Ottawa.

___. 2003. *A Statistical Profile on the Health of First Nations in Canada*. Ottawa: First Nations and Inuit Health Branch. <http://www.hc-sc.gc.ca/fniah-spnia/pubs/ aborig-autoch/2009-stats-profil/index-eng.php>.

Health Canada. 1998. Taking Action on Population Health: A Position Paper for Health Promotion and Programs Branch Staff. Ottawa: Health Canada.

Health Council of Canada. 2005. *The Health Status of Canada's First Nations, Métis and Inuit Peoples—A Background Paper to Accompany Health Care Renewal in Canada: Accelerating Change*. Toronto: Health Council of Canada.

Health Disparities Task Group of the Federal/Provincial/Territorial Advisory Committee on Population Health and Health Security. 2004. "Reducing Health Disparities – Roles of the health Sector: Discussion Paper." Ottawa: Public Health Agency of Canada.

Heidenheimer, A.J. 1990. "Perspectives on the Perception of Corruption." In A.J. Heidenheimer, M. Johnston and V.T. Le Vine (eds.), *Political Corruption: A Handbook*. New Brunswick, NJ: Transaction Publishers.

Held, D. 1989. *Political Theory and the Modern State: Essays on State, Power and Democracy*. Stanford: Stanford University Press.

Henderson, J.Y. 2007. *Indigenous Diplomacy and the Rights of Peoples: Achieving UN Recognition*. Saskatoon, SK: Purich Press.

Henry, F., C. Tater, W. Mattis and T. Rees. 2000. *The Color of Democracy: Racism in Canadian Society*. Toronto: Harcourt Canada.

Herman, J. 1997. *Trauma and Recovery: The Aftermath of Violence—from Domestic Abuse to Political Terror* (second ed.). New York: Basic Books.

___. 1992. *Trauma and Recovery: The Aftermath of Violence—from Domestic Abuse to Political Terror* (first ed.). New York: Basic Books.

Herman, P.E. 2004. "Introduction: The Resistance to Historicizing Theory." In P.E. Herman (Ed.), *Historicizing Theory*. New York: State University of New York Press.

Hertzman, C. 2000. "The Case for an Early Childhood Development Strategy." *Isuma* Autumn.

____. 1999. "The Biological Embedding of Early Experience and its Effects on Health in Adulthood." *Annals of the New York Academy of Sciences* 896.

____. 1994. *The Lifelong Impact of Childhood Experiences: A Population Health Perspective.* Toronto: Canadian Institute for Advanced Research.

Hess, D.J. 2004. "Medical Modernization, Scientific Research Fields and the Epistemic Politics of Health Social Movements." *Sociology of Health and Illness* 26(6).

Hill, D.M. 2003. *Traditional Medicine in Contemporary Contexts: Protecting and Respecting Indigenous Knowledge and Medicine.* Ottawa, ON: National Aboriginal Health Organization.

Hill, G., W. Forbes, J-M. Berthelot, J. Lindsay and I. McDowell. 1996. "Dementia Among Seniors." Ottawa: Statistics Canada. *Health Reports* 8(2).

Hinkle, E. 1987. "Stress and Disease: The Concept After 50 Years." *Social Science and Medicine* 25.

Hochschild, J. 1981. *What's Fair? American Beliefs about Distributive Justice.* Cambridge: Harvard University Press.

Hoffman, Harlan, and Klabunde. 2003. "Racial Differences in Clinically Localized Treatment for Prostate Cancer." *Medscape News* 11(11). At <http://www.medscape.com/viewarticle/462914>.

Hofrichter, R. (ed.). 2003. *Health and Social Justice: Politics, Ideology and Inequity in the Distribution of Disease.* San Francisco: Jossey-Bass.

Hollinsworth, D. 1998. *Race & Racism in Australia* (second ed.). Riverwood, AU: Social Science Press.

Hou, F., and G. Picot. 2003a. "The Rise of Low Income Rates Among Immigrants in Canada." Analytical Studies Branch Research Paper, 198. Ottawa: Statistics Canada.

____. 2003b. "Visible-minority Neighbourhood Enclaves: Labour Market Outcomes of Immigrants." In C. Beach, A. Green and J. Reitz (eds.), *Canadian Immigration Policy for the 21st Century.* Kingston, ON: John Deutsch Institute.

Houston, M., and J.T. Wood. 1996. "Difficult Dialogues, Expanded Horizons: Communicating across Race and Class." In J.T. Wood (ed.), *Gendered Relationships.* Mountainview, CA: Mayfield Publishing.

Howitt, R. 1996 *Resources, Nations and Indigenous peoples.* Melbourne: Oxford University Press.

Howlett, M., and M. Ramesh. 2003. *Studying Public Policy: Policy Cycles and Policy Subsystems.* Oxford: Oxford University Press.

HSF (Heart and Stroke Foundation of Canada). 2009. *Statistics: Heart and Stroke Foundation of Canada.* Ottawa: Author

____. 2007. *Time to Bridge the Gender Gap.* Ottawa.

Hulchanski, D. 2007. "The Three Cities within Toronto: Income Polarization Among Toronto's Neighbourhoods 1970–2000." Toronto: University of Toronto Centre for Urban Community Studies. *Research Bulletin* 41.

Human Rights and Equal Opportunity Commission. 1991. *Racist Violence: Report of the National Inquiry into Racist Violence in Australia.* Canberra: Australian Government Printing Service.

Humphery, Y.K. 2001. "Dirty Questions: Indigenous Health and 'Western Research.'"

Australia and New Zealand Journal of Public Health 25(3).

Hunt, P. 2007. *Report of the Special Rapporteur on the Right of Everyone to the Highest Standard of Physical and Mental Health.* United Nations General Assembly, New York, January 17 (A/HRC/2/28). <ohchr.org>.

Hwang, S., and A. Bugeja. 2000. "Barriers to Appropriate Diabetes Management Among Homeless People in Toronto." *Canadian Medical Association Journal* 163(2).

Hyman, I. 2007. *Immigration and Health: Reviewing Evidence of the Healthy Immigrant Effect in Canada.* CERIS Working Paper No. 55. Toronto: Joint Centre of Excellence for Research on Immigration and Settlement.

Illich, I. 1976. *Limits to Medicine, Medical Nemesis: The Expropriation of Health.* Middlesex, England: Penguin Books.

Innocenti Research Centre. 2008. *The Child Care Transition: A League Table of Early Childhood Education and Care in Economically Advanced Countries.* Florence: Innocenti Research Centre.

___. 2007. *An Overview of Child Well-being in Rich Countries: A Comprehensive Assessment of the Lives and Well-being of Children and Adolescents in the Economically Advanced Nations.* Florence Italy: Innocenti Research Centre.

Institute of Population and Public Health. 2003. *The Future of Public Health in Canada: Developing a Public Health System for the 21st Century.* Toronto: Institute of Population and Public Health.

Ioannidis, J.P., E.E. Ntzani and T.A. Trikalinos. 2004. "'Racial' Differences in Genetic Effects for Complex Diseases." *Nature Genetics* 36.

Jackson, A. 2000. "Taxes, Growth and Inequality." *Behind the Numbers: Economic Facts, Figures and Analysis* 2(4). Ottawa: Canadian Center for Policy Alternatives.

Jakubowski, L. 1997. *Immigration and the Legalization of Racism.* Halifax: Fernwood Publishing.

James, C. 1996. *Perspectives on Racism and the Human Services Sector.* Toronto: University of Toronto Press.

Jang, Y., J.A. Mortimer, W.E. Haly and A.B. Graves. 2004. "The Role of Social Engagement in Life Satisfaction: Its Significance Among older Individuals with Disease and Disability." *Journal of Applied Gerontology* 23.

Jenson, J., and M. Papillon. 2001. *The Changing Boundaries of Citizenship. A Review and a Research Agenda.* Canadian Policy Research Networks.

Johnstone, M.J., and O. Kanitsaki. 2010. "The Neglect of Racism as an Ethical Issue in Health Care." *Journal of Immigrant and Minority Health* 12(4).

Jolanki, O. 2004. "Moral Argumentation in Talk About Health and Old Age." *Health: An Interdisciplinary Journal for the Social Study of Health, Illness and Medicine* 8(4).

Jones, C. 2002. "Unequal Treatment: Confronting Racial and Ethnic Disparities in Heath Care." March 20. National Academy of Sciences Institute of Medicine Report.

___. 2000. "Levels of Racism: A Theoretical Framework and a Gardener's Tale." *American Journal of Public Health* 90.

Jones, J., S. and Pugh. 2005. "Ageing Gay Men: Lessons from the Sociology of Embodiment." *Men & Masculinities* 7(3).

Kafele, K. 2004. "Racial Discrimination and Mental Health: Racialized and Aboriginal

Communities." <ohrc.on.ca/en/issues/racism/racepolicydialogue/kk>.

Kane, M.N. 2008. "Imagining Recovery, Resilience, and Vulnerability at 75: Percpetions of Social Work Students." *Educational Gerontology* 34.

Kaplan, G. 2009. *The Poor Pay More: Poverty's High Cost to Health.* Ann Arbor, MI: University of Michigan Center for Social Epidemiology and Population Health.

Karlsen, S., and J.Y. Nazroo. 2002. "Relation Between Racial Discrimination, Social Class, and Health Among Ethnic Minority Groups." *American Journal of Public Health* 92(4).

Kauffman, J.S., and R.S. Cooper. 1996. "Descriptive Studies of Racial Differences in Disease: In Search of the Hypothesis." *Public Health Reports* 110.

Kawachi, I., B.P. Kennedy and R.G. Wilkinson. 2000. *Income Inequality and Health* (second ed.). New York: New Press.

Kerstetter, S. 2002. *Rags and Riches: Wealth Inequality in Canada.* Ottawa: Canadian Centre for Policy Alternatives.

Kim, J., K.T. Ashing-Giwa, M. Kagawa-Singer and J.S. Tejero. 2006. "Breast Cancer Among Asian Americans: Is Acculturation Related to Health-Related Quality of Life?" *Oncology Nursing Forum* 33(6).

Kimlin, T.A., G. Padilla and J. Tejero. 2004. "Understanding the Breast Cancer Experience of Latina and Caucasian Cancer Survivors." *Psychooncology* 13.

Kingdon, J.W. 2001. "A Model of Agenda-setting, with Applications." *Law Review* 2.

____. 1995. *Agenda, Alternatives, and Public Policies* (second ed.). New York: HarperCollins.

Kira, I. . 2001. "Taxonomy of Trauma and Trauma Assessment." *Traumatology* 7(2).

Kirkpatrick, S., L. and McIntyre. 2009. "The Chief Public Health Officer's Report on Health Inequalities: What are the Implications for Public Health Practitioners and Researchers?" *Canadian Journal of Public Health* 100(2).

Knudsen, J.C. 1995. "When Trust Is on Trial: Negotiating Refugee Narratives." In D. Valentine and J. Knudsen (eds.), *Mistrusting Refugees.* Berkeley: University of California Press.

Kofman, E. 2004. "Gendered Global Migrations: Diversity and Stratification." *International Feminist Journal of Politics* 6(4).

Krieger, N. 2005. "Introduction." *Health Disparities and the Body Politic.* Harvard School of Public Health Symposium Series. Boston: Harvard University. <bvsde. paho.org/bvsacd/cd56/disparities.pdf>.

____. 2003. "Does Racism Harm Health? Did Child Abuse Exist before 1962? On Explicit Questions, Critical Science, and Current Controversies: An Ecosocial Perspective." *American Journal of Public Health* 93(2).

____. 2001a. "Theories for Social Epidemiology: An Ecosocial Perspective." *International Journal of Epidemiology* 30.

____. 2001b. "A Glossary of Social Epidemiology." *Epidemiological Bulletin* 23(1). <http://www.paho.org/english/sha/be_v23n1-glossary.htm>.

____. 1999. "Embodying Inequality: A Review of Concepts, Measures, and Methods for Studying Health Consequences of Discrimination." *International Journal of Health Services* 29(2).

____. 1987. "Shades of Difference: Theoretical Underpinnings of the Medical Controversy on Black-White Differences, 1830–1870." *International Journal of Health Services* 17.

Krieger, N., D.L. Rowley, A.A. Herman, B. Avery and M.T. Phillips. 1993. "Racism, Sexism, and Social Class: Implications for Studies of Health, Disease, and Well-being." *American Journal of Preventive Medicine* 9(6).

Krug, E., J. Mercy, L. Dahlberg and A. Zwi. 2009. "The World Report on Violence and Health." *The Lancet* 360(9339).

Kuhn, T.S. 1970. *The Structure of Scientific Revolutions*. Chicago: University of Chicago Press.

Kunitz, S.J. 1994. *Disease and Social Diversity: The European Impact on the Health of Non-Europeans*. New York: Oxford University Press.

Kuran, H.J. 2002. *The Barriers to Healthy Living and Movement for Frail Aboriginal Elders*. Kahnawake, QC: National Indian and Inuit Community Health Representatives Organization. <niichro.com/cfc/cfc_3.html>.

Labonte, R., and S. Penfold. 1981. "Canadian Perspectives in Health Promotion: A Critique." *Health Education* 19.

Lake, S. 2010. *Willem de Kooning: The Artist's Materials*. Los Angeles: Getty Conservation Institute.

Langille, D. 2008. "Follow the Money: How Business and Politics Shape our Health." In D. Raphael (ed.), *Social Determinants of Health: Canadian Perspectives* (second ed.). Toronto: Canadian Scholars Press.

Lantz, P.M., J.S. House, J.M. Lepkowski, D.R. Williams, R.P. Mero and J.J. Chen. 1998. "Socioeconomic Factors, Health Behaviors, and Mortality." *Journal of the American Medical Association* 279(21).

Lattas, A. 2001. "Redneck Thought: Racism, Guilt and Aborigines." *UTS Review* 7.

Lavis, J. 2002. "Ideas at the Margin or Marginalized Ideas? Nonmedical Determinants of Health in Canada." *Health Affairs* 21(2).

Laws, G. 1995. "Understanding Ageism: Lessons from Feminism and Postmodernism." *The Gerontologist* 35(1).

LEAF (Legal Action and Education Fund). 2010. *About LEAF*. Ottawa: LEAF. <http://leaf.ca/about-leaf/>.

____. 2004. *The Court Challenges Program*. Ottawa: LEAF. <leaf.ca/>.

____. 1990. *Albrecht v. Albrecht*. Ottawa: LEAF. <http://leaf.ca/cases/albrecht-v-albrecht/>.

Lee, M. 2007. *Eroding Tax Fairness: Tax Incidence in Canada, 1998 to 2005*. Ottawa: Canadian Centre for Policy Alternatives.

Leenen, F., J. Dumais, N. McInnis, P. Turton, L. Stratychuk, M. Bemeth et al. 2008. "The Political Economy of Health." International People's Health University. <iphu.org/en/polecon>.

Legowski, B., and L. McKay. 2000. "Health Beyond Health Care: Twenty-five Years of Federal Health Policy Development." CPRN Discussion Paper No. H|04. Ottawa: Canadian Policy Research Networks (CPRN).

Lemstra, M., C. Neudorf and J. Opondo. 2006. "Health Disparity by Neighbourhood Income." *Canadian Journal of Public Health* 97(6).

Lessa, I. 2006. "Discursive Struggles Within Social Welfare: Restaging Teen Motherhood." *British Journal of Social Work* 36(2).

Lewchuk, W., A. de Wolff, A. King and M. Polyani. 2003. "From Job Strain to Employment Strain: Health Effects of Precarious Employment." *Just Labours* 3.

Leys, C. 2001. *Market-Driven Politics*. London, UK: Verso.

Li, P. 2001. "The Racial Subtext in Canada's Immigration Discourse." *Journal of International Migration and Integration* 2(1).

Li, W.H., and L.A. Sadler. 1991. "Low Nucleotide Diversity in Man." *Genetics* 129.

Lightman, E., A. Mitchell and B. Wilson. 2008. *Poverty Is Making Us Sick: A Comprehensive Survey of Income and Health in Canada.* Toronto: Community Social Planning Council of Toronto and Wellesley Institute.

Lindsay, C., and M Almey. 2006. "Immigrant Women." In *Women in Canada: A Gender-Based Statistical Report,* (fifth ed.). Ottawa: Statistics Canada <http://www.statcan.gc.ca/pub/89-503-x/89-503-x2005001-eng.pdf>.

Lippman, A. 1993. "Prenatal Genetic Testing and Geneticization: Mother Matters for All." *Fetal Diagnosis and Therapy* 8(1).

Lipset, S.M. 1996. *American Exceptionalism: A Double-Edged Sword.* New York: W.W. Norton.

Lipsky, M. 1980. *Street-Level Bureaucracy: Dilemmas of the Individual in Public Services.* New York: Russell Sage Foundation.

Llácer, A., M. Zunzunegui, J. del Amo, L. Mazarrasa and F. Bolumar. 2007. "The Contribution of a Gender Perspective to the Understanding of Migrants' Health." *Journal of Epidemiology and Community Health* 61(II).

Logan, S.M.L., E.M. Freeman and R.G. McRoy (eds.). 1990. *Social Work Practice with Black Families: A Culturally Specific Perspective.* NY: Longman.

Lopez, I.F.H. 1994. "The Social Construction of Race: Some Observations on Illusion, Fabrication, and Choice." *Harvard Civil Rights-Civil Liberties Law Review* 29: 1–62. <http://www.law.berkeley.edu/php-programs/faculty/facultyPubsPDF.php?facID=301&pubID=9>.

Lovell, A. 2009. "Racism, Poverty and Inner City Health: Current Knowledge and Practices." Unpublished Doctoral dissertation, Queen's University.

Lux, M.L. 2001. *Medicine That Walks: Disease Medicine and Canadian Plains Native People 1880–1940.* Toronto: University of Toronto Press.

Macarov, D. 2003. *What the Market Does to People: Privatization, Globalization, and Poverty.* Atlanta GA: Clarity Press.

Macdonald, J. 2004. "Primary Health Care: A Global Overview." *Primary Health Care Research & Development* 5(4).

Macinko, J., H. Montenagro and C. Nebot. 2007. "Renewing Primary Health Care in the Americas: A Position Paper of the Pan American Health Organization/World Health Organization (PAHO/WHO)." Washington, DC: PAHO.

Macionis, J.J., and L.M. Gerber 2005. *Sociology.* Toronto: Pearson.

Macklin, A. 1994. "On the Inside Looking In: Foreign Domestic Workers in Canada." In W. Giles and S. Arat-Koç (eds.), *Maid in the Market: Women's Paid Domestic Labour.* Halifax: Fernwood Publishing.

Maliski, S.L., S. Connor, A. Fink and M.S. Litwin. 2006. "Information Desired and Acquired by Men with Prostate Cancer: Data from Ethnic Focus Groups." *Health Education & Behavior* 33(3).

Mann, J.M., S. Griskin, M.H. Grodin and G.J. Annas. 1999. *Health and Human Rights: A Reader.* New York: Routledge.

Mar'i, S.K. 1988. "Challenges to Minority Counselling: Arabs in Israel." *International Journal of the Advancement of Counselling* 11(1).

Marmot, M. 2008. "Michael Marmot on Eliminating Social Injustice in Health." *Health*

Service Journal October 30. <hsj.co.uk/michael-marmot-on-eliminating-social-injustice-in-health/1901424.article>.

Marmot, M., and R. Wilkinson. 1999. *The Social Determinants of Health.* New York: Oxford University Press.

Martin, R. 2006. "Patient Power, Human Rights and Access to Primary Health Care Services in an NHS System." *Primary Health Care Research and Development* 5(3).

Marx, K. 1977 [1845]. *A Contribution to the Critique of Political Economy,* Moscow: Progress Publishers.

Mayer, C.S. 1987. *In Search of Stability: Explorations in Historical Political Economy.* Cambridge: Cambridge University Press.

McBride, S., and J. Shields. 1997. *Dismantling a Nation: The Transition to Corporate Rule in Canada.* Halifax, Canada: Fernwood Publishing.

McCorquodale, J.C. 1997. "Aboriginal Identity: Legislative, Judicial and Administrative Definitions." *Australian Aboriginal Studies* 2: 24–35.

McDonald, M., and C. Quell. 2008. "Bridging the Common Divide: The Importance of Both 'Cohesion' and 'Inclusion.'" *Canadian Diversity/Diversité Canadienne* 6(2).

McGibbon, E. 2009. "Health and Health Care: A Human Rights Perspective." In D. Raphael (ed.), *Social Determinants of Health* (second ed.). Toronto, ON: Canadian Scholars' Press.

____. 2008. "Barriers in Access to Health Services for Rural Aboriginal and African Canadians: A Scoping Review." Canadian Institutes for Health Research Scoping Review Symposium: Keynote address notes: 'Improving Access for Vulnerable and Underserved Populations.' Ottawa, ON, January.

____. 2007. "The Social Determinants of Health: When Care is Political." Keynote address notes, Canadian Association of Rehabilitation Professionals Atlantic Conference, Moncton, NB, September.

____. 2004. "Towards a Reformulation of the Nature of Stress in Nursing: An Institutional Ethnography." Unpublished Doctoral dissertation. Toronto: University of Toronto.

McGibbon, E., A. Calliste, E. Arbuthnot, R. Bassett, C. Cameron, H. Graham et al. 2008. "Barriers in Access to Health Services for Rural Aboriginal and African Canadians." Research report, Canadian Institutes for Health Research, Ottawa.

McGibbon, E., P. Didham, D. Smith, M. Malaudzi, A. Sochan and S. Barton. 2009. *Decolonization of Nursing Education: A Paradigm Shift for the New Millennium.* Book of abstracts published from the Proceedings of the Canadian Association of Schools of Nursing National Conference, Moncton, NB, May.

McGibbon, E., and J. Etowa. 2009. *Anti-Racist Health Care Practice.* Toronto: Canadian Scholar's Press.

____. 2007. "Health Inequities and the Social Determinants of Health: Spatial Contexts of Oppression." Invited keynote presentation, Nova Scotia Health Research Foundation Health Geomatics Conference, Halifax, NS, October.

McGibbon, E., J. Etowa and C. McPherson. 2008a. "Health Care Access as a Social Determinant of Health." *Canadian Nurse Journal* 104(7).

____. 2008b. *Health as a Human Right: The Role of Mixed Methods Research in Global Justice.* Book of abstracts published from the Proceedings of the Fourth International Congress of Qualitative Inquiry, University of Illinois, Urbana, Illinois, May.

McGibbon, E., and C. McPherson. 2011. "Applying Intersectionality Theory and Complexity Theory to Address the Social Determinants of Women's Health." *Women's Health and Urban Life: An International Journal* (10) 1. University of Toronto Press.

McIntyre, L. 2004. "Food Insecurity." In D. Raphael (ed.), *Social Determinants of Health: Canadian Perspectives*. Toronto: Canadian Scholars' Press.

McIntyre, L., N.T. Glanville, S. Officer, B. Anderson, K.D. Raine and J.B. Dayle. 2002. "Food Insecurity of Low-Income Lone Mothers and their Children in Atlantic Canada." *Canadian Journal of Public Health* 93.

McIntyre, L., F. Wien, S. Rudderham, L. Etter, C. Moore and N. MacDonald. 2001. *An Exploration of the Stress Experience of Mi'kmaq On-reserve Female Youth in Nova Scotia*. Halifax, NS: Maritime Center of Excellence for Women's Health.

McKeown, D., K. MacCon, N. Day, P. Fleiszer, S. Scott and S.A. Wolfe. 2008. *The Unequal City: Income and Health Inequalities in Toronto*. Toronto: Toronto Public Health.

McKinley, J.B 1975. *The Political Economy of Health*. London: Pluto Press.

McMullin, J. 2008. *Understanding Social Inequality: Intersections of Class, Age, Gender, Ethnicity and Race in Canada* (second ed.). Toronto: Oxford University Press.

McPherson, C., A. Kothari and S. Sibbald. 2010. "Quality Improvement in Primary Health Care in Ontario: An Environmental Scan and Capacity Map." Final report prepared for the Quality Improvement in Primary Healthcare Project and Primary Health Care System Program. <http://www.qiip.ca/user_files/environmentalscan.pdf>.

McPherson, C., and E. McGibbon. 2010a. "Rural Interprofessional Primary Health Care Team Development and Sustainability: Establishing a Research Agenda." *Primary Health Care Research &* Development 11(4).

____. 2010b. "Addressing the Determinants of Child Mental Health: Using Intersectionality to Guide Primary Health Care Renewal." *Canadian Journal of Nursing Research* 42(3).

McPherson, C., J. Popp and R. Lindstrom. 2006. "Reexamining the Paradox of Structure: A Child Health Network Perspective." *Healthcare Papers* 7(2).

McPherson, C., and J. Shamian. 2010. *The Role of Nursing & Midwifery in Primary Health Care Renewal: A Strategic Policy Advisory Report to the WHO Global Advisory Group for Nursing and Midwifery*. Geneva: WHO, Office of Nursing and Midwifery.

McQuaig, L. 1993. *The Wealthy Banker's Wife: The Assault of Equality in Canada*. Toronto: Penguin.

____. 1987. *Behind Closed Doors: How the Rich Won Control of Canada's Tax System —And Ended Up Richer*. Toronto: Viking.

Meadows, L.M., W.E. Thurston and C. Melton. 2001. "Immigrant Women's Health." *Social Science & Medicine* 52(9).

Meany, M.J., M. Szyf and J.R. Seckl. 2007. "Epigenetic Mechanisms of Perinatal Programming of Hypothalamic-Pituitary, Adrenal Function and Health." *Trends in Nuclear Medicine* 13(7).

Mederios, D.M., M. Seehaus, J. Elliot and A. Melaney. 2004. "Providing Mental Health Services for LGBT Teens in a Community Adolescent Health Clinic." *Journal of Gay and Lesbian Psychotherapy* 8(3/4).

Mellor D. 2003. "Contemporary Racism in Australia: The Experiences of Aborigines." *Personality & Social Psychology Bulletin* 29.

Memmi A. 1969. *Dominated Man: Notes Toward a Portrait*. Boston: Beacon Press.

Meng, Y.Y., R.P. Rull, M. Wilhelm, C. Lombardi, J. Balmes and B. Ritz. 2010. "Outdoor Air Pollution and Uncontrolled Asthma in the San Joaquin Valley, California." *Journal of Epidemiology and Community Health* 64(2).

Merkin, S.S., S. Stevenson and N. Powe. 2002. "Geographic Socioeconomic Status, Race, and Advanced-stage Breast Cancer in New York City." *American Journal of Public Health* 92(1).

Mettlin, C., G. Murphy, M. Cunningham and H. Menck. 1997. "The National Cancer Database Report on Race, Age, and Region Variations in Prostate Cancer Treatment." *Cancer* 80.

Mikkonen, J., and D. Raphael. 2010. *Social Determinants of Health: The Canadian Facts*. Toronto: York University. <thecanadianfacts.org/>.

Miles, R., and M. Brown. 2003. *Racism*. London: Routledge.

Mills, S. 1997. *Discourse*. London: Routledge.

Minsky, A. 2009. "Aboriginal Children's Health Below National Averages: United Nations." Innocenti Children's Emergency Fund (UNICEF). *Canwest News Service* June 24.

Morgan, S. 2006. "Pharmaceutical Research and Policy." CIHR Institute of Health Services and Policy Research. *Research Spotlight* August.

Morrison, L., and J. L'Heureux. 2001. "Suicide and Gay/Lesbian/Bisexual Youth: Implications for Clinicians." *Journal of Adolescence* 24.

Mulhall A. 1996. "Cultural Discourse and the Myth of Stress in Nursing and Medicine." *International Journal of Nursing Studies* 33.

Muntaner, C., W.W. Eaton, R. Miech and P. O'Campo. 2004. "Socioeconomic Position and Major Mental Disorders." *Epidemiological Review* 26.

Muntaner, C., and J. Lynch. 2001. "Income Inequality, Social Cohesion, and Class Relations: A Critique of Wilkinson's Neo-Durkheimian Research Program." In Vincent Navarro (ed.), *The Political Economy of Social Inequalities*. New York: Baywood Publishing.

Murray, S., R. Rudd, I. Kirsch, K. Yamamoto and S. Grenier. 2007. *Health Literacy in Canada: Initial Results from the International Adult Literacy Skills Survey*. Ottawa: Canadian Council on Learning.

Mwape, L., A. Sikwese, A. Kapungwe, J. Mwanza, A. Flisher, C. Lund et al. 2010. "Integrating Mental Health into Primary Health Care in Zambia: A Care Provider's Perspective." *International Journal of Mental Health Systems* 4(21).

NAPO (National Anti-Poverty Organization). 2005. *Election Sheet on Poverty in Canada*. December.

National Advisory Council on Aging. 2006. *Seniors in Canada 2006 Report Card*. Ottawa: Government of Canada.

National Health Committee. 1998. *The Social, Cultural and Economic Determinants of Health in New Zealand: Action to Improve Health*. Wellington, NZ: National Health Committee.

Navarro, V. 2009. "What We Mean by Social Determinants of Health." *Global Health Promotion* 16(1).

___. 2007a. "What Is National Health Policy?" *International Journal of Health Services* 37(1).

___. 2007b. "Neoliberalism as Class Ideology: Or the Political Causes of the Growth of Inequalities." *International Journal of Health Services* 37(1).

___. 2002a. "A Historical Review (1965–1997) of Studies on Class, Health, and Quality of Life: A Personal Account." In V. Navaro (ed.), *The Political Economy of Social Inequalities: Consequences for Health and Quality of Life.* New York: Baywood Publishing Company.

___. 2002b. *The Political Economy of Social Inequalities: Consequences for Health and Quality of Life.* New York: Baywood Publishing.

Navarro, V., C. Borrell, J. Benach, C. Muntaner, A. Quiroga, M. Rodrigues-Sanz et al. 2004. "The Importance of the Political and the Social in Explaining Mortality Differentials among the Countries of the OECD, 1950–1998." In V. Navarro (ed.), *The Political and Social Contexts of Health.* Amityville, NY: Baywood Press.

Navarro, V., C. Muntaner, J. Benach, A. Quiroga, M. Rodriguez-Sanz, N. Verges et al. 2006. "Politics and Health Outcomes." *The Lancet* 368: 1–5.

Navarro, V., and L. Shi. 2002. "The Political Context of Social Inequalities and Health." In V. Navarro (ed.), *The Political Economy of Social Inequalities: Consequences for Health and Quality of Life.* Amityville, NY: Baywood.

___. 2001. "The Political Context of Social Inequalities and Health." *International Journal of Health Services* 31(1).

NEADA (National Energy Assistance Director's Association). 2008. *National Energy Assistance Directors' Association Status of State Low Income Heat Energy Assistance Program Funding: State Survey.* Washington, DC.

Neufeld, A., M. Harrison, K. Hughes, M. Stewart and D.L. Spitzer. 2002. "Immigrant Women: Making Connections to Community Resources for Support in Family Caregiving." *Qualitative Health Research* 12(6).

Ng, E., R. Wilkins, F. Gendron and J-M. Berthelot. 2005. *Dynamics of Immigrants' Health in Canada: Evidence from the National Population Health Survey.* Ottawa: Statistics Canada.

Nguyenlo, M., M. Ugarte, I. Fuller, G. Haas and R.K. Portenoy. 2005. "Access to Care for Chronic Pain: Racial and Ethnic Differences." *The Journal of Pain* 6(5).

Niggle, C.J. 1998. "Equality, Democracy, Institutions, and Growth." *Journal of Economic Issues* 32.

Nygren-Krug, H. 2008. "Health and Human Rights: In 25 Questions and Answers." In M. Masellis, S. William and A. Green (eds.), *Concepts and Practice of Humanitarian Medicine.* New York: SpringerLink.

O'Loughlin. 2001. "What Approaches Have Been Used to Foster Healthy Lifestyles and Are They Effective?" <phac-aspc.gc.ca/ph-sp/docs/healthy-sain/chap3-eng.php>.

Oakley-Girvan, I., L. Kolonel, R. Gallagher, A. Wu, A. Felberg and A. Whittemore. 2003. "Stage at Diagnosis and Survival in a Multiethnic Cohort of Prostate Cancer Patients." *American Journal of Public Health* 93(10).

OECD (Organization for Economic Co-operation and Development). 2009. *Society at a Glance: Social Indicators 2009.* Paris: Organisation for Economic Co-operation and Development.

___. 2008. *Growing Unequal: Income Distribution and Poverty in OECD Nations.* Paris: Organization for Economic Co-operation and Development.

___. 2007a. *Health at a Glance: OECD Iindicators 2007.* Paris: Organization for

Economic Cooperation and Development.

___. 2007b. *Society at a Glance 2006, OECD Social Indicators*. Paris: Organization for Economic Co-operation and Development.

Oliver, M.N., and C. Muntaner. 2005. "Researching Health Inequities Among African Americans: The Imperative to Understand Social Class." *International Journal of Health Services* 35(3).

Ontario Human Rights Commission. 1992. *Ontario Human Rights Code Review Task Force*. Ottawa: Ontario Human Rights Commission.

OPHA (Ontario Public Health Association). 2010. *Understanding the Role of Public Health in Chronic Disease Prevention in Ontario*. Ottawa.

Ornstein, M. 2000. *Ethno-Racial Inequality in the City of Toronto: An Analysis of the 1996 Census*. Toronto: Access and Equity Unit, Strategic and Corporate Policy Division, Chief Administrator's Office.

Orpana, H.M., L. Lemyre and R. Gravel. 2007. "Income and Psychological Distress: The Role of the Social Environment." *Health Reports* 20(1).

Overall, C. 2006. "Old Age and Ageism, Impairment and Ableism: Exploring the Conceptual and Material Connections." *National Women's Studies Association Journal* 18(1).

Overbeek, H., and K. van der Pijl. 1993. "Restructuring Capital and Restructuring Hegemony: Neoliberalism and the Unmaking of the Post-War Order." In H. Overbeek (ed.), *Restructuring Hegemony in the Global Political Economy*. London: Routledge.

Page, H., and T. Thomas. 1994. "White Public Space and the Constructions of White Privilege in U.S. Health Care: Fresh Concepts." *Medical Anthropology Quarterly* 8(1).

Pal, L. 2006. *Beyond Policy Analysis: Public Issue Management in Turbulent Times*. Toronto: Nelson.

Paradies, Y. 2007. "Racism." In B. Carson, T. Dunbar and R. D. Chenhall (eds.), *An Introduction to International Health*. Crows Nest, NSW, AU: Allen and Unwin.

___. 2006a. "Defining, Conceptualising and Characterizing Racism in Health Research." *Critical Public Health* 16(2).

___. 2006b. "A Review of Psychosocial Stress and Chronic Disease for 4th World Indigenous Peoples and African Americans." *Ethnicity and Disease* 16(1): 295–308.

Paul, D. 2006. *We Were Not the Savages*. Halifax: Fernwood Publishing.

Pederson, A., and D. Raphael. 2006. "Gender, Race, and Health." In D. Raphael, T. Bryant and M. Rioux (eds.), *Staying Alive: Critical Perspectives on Health, Illness, and Health Care*. Toronto: Canadian Scholars Press.

Pedersen, A., I. Walker and M. Wise. 2005. "'Talk Does Not Cook Rice': Beyond Anti-Racism Rhetoric to Strategies for Social Action." *The Australian Psychologist* 40.

Penard-Morand, C., C. Raherison, D. Charpin, C. Kopferschmitt, F. Lavaud, D. Caillaud et al. 2010. "Long-Term Exposure to Close-Proximity Air Pollution and Asthma and Allergies in Urban Children." *European Respirology Journal* 36.

Periago, M.R. 2007. "Renewing Primary Health Care in the Americas: The Pan American Health Organization Proposal for the Twenty-first Century." <http://journal.paho.org/uploads/1178725284.pdf>.

___. 2004. *Women Bear Burden of Home Care*. Pan American Health Organization World Health Organization. 2004. Press release, March 8. Washington, DC.

Petras, J., and S. Vieux. 1992. "Twentieth Century Neoliberals: Inheritors of the Exploits of Columbus." *Latin American Perspectives* 19(3).

Pieterse, A.L., and R.T. Carter. 2007. "An Examination of the Relationship Between General Life Stress, Racism-related Stress and Psychological Health Among Black Men." *Journal of Counseling Psychology* 54(1).

Potvin, L., L. Richard and A. Edwards. 2000. "Knowledge of Cardiovascular Disease Risk Factors among the Canadian Population: Relationships with Indicators of Socioeconomic Status." *Canadian Medical Association Journal* 162.

Poudrier, J., and R.T. Mac-Lean. 2009. "'We've Fallen Into the Cracks': Aboriginal Women's Experiences with Breast Cancer through Photovoice." *Nursing Inquiry* 16(4).

Preibisch, K. 2005. "Gender Transformative Odysseys: Tracing the Experiences of Transnational Migrant Women in Rural Canada." *Canadian Women's Studies* 24(4).

Presser, S. 2008. *Heat or Eat: Energy Insecurity in New Jersey*. Newark: Association for Children of New Jersey.

Pressman, J.L., and A. Wildavsky. 1984. *Implementation: How Great Expectations in Washington Are Dashed in Oakland* (third ed.). Berkeley, CA: University of California Press.

Prilletensky, I., and L. Gonick. 1996. "Politics Change, Oppression Remains: On the Psychology and Politics of Oppression." *Political Psychology* 17(1).

Pruegger, V. 2009. *Inequality in Calgary: The Racialization of Poverty*. Calgary: City of Calgary.

Public Health Agency of Canada. 2008a. *Social and Economic Factors that Influence Our Health and Contribute to Health Inequalities: The Chief Public Health Officer's Report on the State of Public Health in Canada*. Ottawa.

___. 2008b. "National Collaborating Centre for Determinants of Health." <nccdh.ca/>.

___. 2007. "Canada's Response to WHO Commission on Social Determinants of Health." <phac-aspc.gc.ca/sdh-dss/bg-eng.php>.

Quan, H., A. Fong, C. De Coster, J. Wang, R. Musto, T.W. Noseworthy and W.A. Ghali. 2006. "Variation in Health Services Utilization Among Ethnic Populations." *Canadian Medical Association Journal* 174(6).

Quick, J.C., D.L. Nelson, J.D. Quick and D.K. Orman. 2001. "An Isomorphic Theory of Stress: The Dynamics of Person-Environment Fit." *Stress and Health* 17.

Radecki, S.E., R.L. Kane, D.H. Solomon, R.C. Mendhall and J.C. Beck. 1988a. "Do Physicians Spend Less Time with Older Patients?" *Journal of the American Geriatrics Society* 36.

___. 1988b. "Are Physicians Sensitive to the Special Problems of Older Patients?" *Journal of the American Geriatrics Society* 36.

Rainville, B., and S. Brink. 2001. "Food Insecurity in Canada, 1998–1999." Research Paper R-01 2E. Ottawa: Applied Research Branch Human Resources Development, Canada.

Rainwater, L., and T.M. Smeeding. 2003. *Poor Kids in a Rich Country: America's Children in Comparative Perspective*. New York: Russell Sage Foundation.

Raphael, D. 2009a. "Social Determinants of Health: An Overview of Key Issues and

Themes." In D, Raphael (ed.), *Social Determinants of Health*. Toronto: Canadian Scholars Press.

___. 2009b. "Escaping from the Phantom Zone: Social Determinants of Health, Public Health Units and Public Policy in Canada." *Health Promotion International* 24(2).

___. 2008a. "Grasping at Straws: A Recent History of Health Promotion in Canada." *Critical Public Health* 18(4).

___ (ed.). 2008b. *Social Determinants of Health: Canadian Perspectives* (second ed.). Toronto: Canadian Scholars' Press.

___. 2007a. "Canadian Public Policy and Poverty in International Perspective." In D. Raphael (ed.), *Poverty and Policy in Canada: Implications for Health and Quality of Life*. Toronto: Canadian Scholars' Press.

___. 2007b. "The Politics of Poverty." In D. Raphael (ed.), *Poverty and Policy in Canada: Implications for Health and Quality of Life*. Toronto: Canadian Scholars' Press.

___. 2006. "Social Determinants of Health: Present Status, Unresolved Questions, and Future Directions." *International Journal of Health Services* 36.

___. 2004. "Strengthening the Social Determinants of Health: The Toronto Charter for a Healthy Canada." In Dennis Raphael (ed.). *The Social Determinants of Health: Canadian Perspectives*. Toronto: Canadian Scholars Press.

___. 2003. "Bridging the Gap Between Knowledge and Action on the Societal Determinants of Cardiovascular Disease: How one Canadian Community Effort Hit — and Hurdled — the Lifestyle Wall." *Health Education* 103.

___. 2002. *Social Justice Is Good for Our Hearts: Why Societal Factors — Not Lifestyles — are Major Causes of Heart Disease in Canada and Elsewhere*. <cwhn.ca/resources/heart_health/justice2.pdf>.

Raphael, D., S. Anstice and K. Raine. 2003. "The Social Determinants of the Incidence and Management of Type 2 Diabetes Mellitus: Are we Prepared to Rethink our Questions and Redirect our Research Activities?" *Leadership in Health Services* 16.

Raphael, D., and T. Bryant. 2006a. *Staying Alive*. Toronto: Canadian Scholar's Press.

___. 2006b. "Public Health Concerns in Canada, the US, the UK, and Sweden." In Dennis Raphael, Toba Bryant and Marcia Rioux (eds.), *Staying Alive: Critical Perspectives on Health, Illness, and Health Care*. Toronto: Canadian Scholar's Press.

___. 2006c. "Maintaining Population Health in a Period of Welfare State Decline: Political Economy as the Missing Dimension in Health Promotion Theory and Practice." *Promotion and Education* 13(4).

Raphael, D., T. Bryant and A. Curry-Stevens. 2009. "Surmounting the Barriers: Making Action on the Social Determinants of Health a Public Policy Priority." In D, Raphael (ed.), *Social Determinants of Health*. Toronto: Canadian Scholars Press.

___. 2004. "Toronto Charter Outlines Future Health Policy Directions for Canada and Elsewhere." *Health Promotion International* 19.

Raphael, D., A. Curry-Stevens and T. Bryant. 2008. "Barriers to Addressing the Social Determinants of Health: Insights from the Canadian Experience." *Health Policy* 88.

Raphael, D., and E.S. Farrell. 2002. "Beyond Medicine and Lifestyle: Addressing the Societal Determinants of Cardiovascular Disease in North America." *Leadership in Health Services* 15.

Raphael, D., J. Macdonald, R. Labonte, R. Colman, K. Hayward and R. Torgerson. 2004. "Researching Income and Income Distribution as a Determinant of Health in Canada: Gaps Between Theoretical Knowledge, Research Practice, and Policy Implementation." *Health Policy* 72.

Restrepo, H.E. 1996. "Introduction." In Pan.American Health Organization (ed.), *Health Promotion: An Anthology*. Washington, DC: Pan American Health Organization.

Reutter, L., M. Steward, G. Veenstra, R. Love, D. Raphael and E. Makwarimba. 2009. "Who Do They Think We Are Anyway? Perceptions of and Responses to Poverty Stigma." *Qualitative Health Research* 19(3).

Ridde, V. 2009. "Policy Implementation in an African State: An Extension of Kingdon's Multiple Streams Approach." *Public Administration* 87(4).

____. 2008a. "Equity and Health Policy in Africa: Using Concept Mapping in Burkina Faso." *BMC Health Service Research* 8: 90.

Robb, C., H. Chen and W.E. Haley. 2002. "Ageism in Mental Health Care: A Critical Review." *Journal of Clinical Geropsychology* 8(1).

Romualdi, C., D. Balding, I.S. Nasidze, G. Risch, M. Robichaux, S.T. Sherry et al. 2002. "Patterns of Human Diversity, Within and Among Continents, Inferred from Biallelic DNA Polymorphisms." *Genome Res* 12.

Rosen, F., and D. McFadyen (eds.). 1995. *Free Trade and Economic Restructuring in Latin America*. New York: Monthly Review Press.

Ross, C.E., and J. Mirowsky. 2001. "Neighborhood Disadvantage, Disorder, and Health." *Journal of Health & Social Behavior* 42(3).

Rotermann, M. 2005. "Seniors' Health Care Use." *Supplement to Health Reports* 16. Statistics Canada, Catalogue 82-003.

Rothenberg, B., T. Pearson, J. Zwanziger and D. Mukamel. 2004. "Explaining Dsparities in Access to High-Quality Cardiac Surgeons." *Annals of Thoracic Surgery* 78(1).

Rottier, R., and N. Jackson. 2003. "Unravelling the Rhetoric of Population Ageing: The Social Construction of "Troubles" and "Issues"—an Australian Perspective." *International Journal of Communication* 13(1–2).

Rowe, J.W. 1990. "Work Ability in Later Life." In R. Butler, M. Oberlink and M. Schechter (eds.), *The Promise of Productive Aging: From Biology to Social Policy*. New York: Springer.

Rowe, J.W., and R.L. Kahn. 1987. "Human Aging: Usual and Successful." *Science* 237.

Roy, J. 2008. "Legalized Racism." Toronto: Canadian Race Relations Foundation. <crr.ca/content/view/224/377/lang,english/>.

Royal Commission on Aboriginal Peoples. 1996. *Report of the Royal Commission on Aboriginal Peoples*. Ottawa: Canada Communication Group.

____. 1995. *Bridging The Cultural Divide: A Report on Aboriginal Peoples and Criminal Justice in Canada*. Ottawa: Canada Communication Group.

Ryff, C.D. 1989. "In the Eyes of the Beholder: Views of Psychological Well-being Among Middle-Aged and Older Adults." *Psychology & Aging* 4.

Said, E.W. 1979. *Orientalism*. New York: Vintage Books.

Saint-Arnaud, S., and P. Bernard. 2003. "Convergence or Resilience? A Hierarchical Cluster Analysis of the Welfare Regimes in Advanced Countries." *Current Sociology* 51(5).

Sanders, C., J. Donovan and P. Dieppe. 2002. "The Significance and Consequences of Having Painful and Disabled Joints in Older Age: Co-existing Accounts of Normal and Disrupted Biographies." *Sociology of Health & Illness* 24(2).

Sapolsky, R.M. 1992. *Stress, the Aging Brain, and Mechanisms of Neuron Death.* Cambridge: MIT Press.

Sarkisian, C.A., R.D. Hays and C.M. Mangione. 2002. "Do Older Adults Expect to Age Successfully? The Association Between Expectations Regarding Aging and Beliefs Regarding Healthcare Seeking Among Older Adults." *Journal of the American Geriatrics Society* 50.

Saunders, R. 2003. *Defining Vulnerability in the Labour Market.* Ottawa: Canadian Policy Research Networks.

Sauvé, J., and M. Burns. 2009. "Residents of Canada's Shelters for Abused Women, 2008." *Juristat* 29(2). Components of Statistics Canada Catalogue no. 85-200-X. Ottawa.

Saxena, S., A. Majeed and M. Jones. 1999. "Socioeconomic Differences in Childhood Consultation Rates in General Practice in England and Wales: Prospective Cohort Study." *British Medical Journal* 318(7184).

Scarth, T. (ed.). 2004. *Hell and High Water: An Assessment of Paul Martin's Record and Implications for the Future.* Ottawa: Canadian Centre for Policy Alternatives.

Scheidt, R.G., D.R. Humpherys and J.B. Yorgason. 1999. "Successful Aging: What's Not to Like?" *Journal of Applied Gerontology* 18.

Schultz, A., D. Williams, B. Israel and L. Lempert. 2002. "Racial and Spatial Relations as Fundamental Determinants of Health in Detroit." *The Milbank Quarterly* 80(4).

Schwartz, A.C., R.L. Bradley, M. Sexton, A. Sherry and K.J. Ressler. 2005. "Posttraumatic Stress Disorder Among African Americans in an Inner City Mental Health Clinic." *Psychiatric Services* 56: 212–15.

Scott, K. 2010. *Community Vitality: A Report of the Institute of Wellbeing.* Vancouver: Institute of Wellbeing.

Seear, M. 2007. *An Introduction to International Health.* Toronto: Canadian Scholars' Press.

Seligman, H.K., A.W. Bindman, E. Vittinghoff, A.M. Kanaya and M.B. Kushel. 2007. "Food Insecurity Is Associated with Diabetes Mellitus: Results from the National Health Examination and Nutrition Examination Survey (NHANES) 1999–2002." *Journal of General Medicine* 22(7).

Senate Subcommittee on Population Health. 2008. *Canada Senate Subcommittee Reports: International Community's Approach to Population Health.* <health-equity.blogspot.com/2008/03/eq-canada-senate-subcommittee-reports.html>.

Shamian, J. 2007. *Home Care: The Unfinished Policy.* Ottawa: Victorian Order of Nurses.

Shapcott, M., and D. Hulchanski. 2004. *Finding Room: Policy Options for a Canadian Rental Housing Strategy.* Toronto: Center for Urban and Community Studies.

Sharpe, P.A. 1995. "Older Women and Health Services." *Women & Health* 22(3).

Shaw, M., D. Dorling, D. Gordon and G.D. Smith. 1999. *The Widening Gap: Health Inequalities and Policy in Britain.* Bristol: Policy Press.

Shelter Cymru. 2004. *Housing and the Asthma Epidemic in Whales.* Shelter Cymru, Swansea, Wales, UK. <sheltercymru.org.uk/images/pdf/HousingandAsthma.pdf>.

Shields, M. 2008. "Community Belonging and Self-perceived Health." *Health Reports* 19(2). Statistics Canada Catalogue no. 82-003, June.

___. 2004. "Social Anxiety Disorder—Beyond Shyness." *Supplement to Health Reports* 15. Statistics Canada Catalogue no. 82-003.

Shields, M., and J. Chen. 1999. "Health Among Older Adults." *Health Reports* 11(3).

Shields, M., and L. Martel. 2005. "Healthy Living Among Seniors." *Supplement to Health Reports* 16. Statistics Canada, Catalogue 82-003.

Sidanius, J. 1993. "The Psychology of Group Conflict and the Dynamics of Oppression: A Social Dominance Perspective." In S. Iyengar and W.J. McGuire (eds.), *Explorations in Political Psychology*. London: Duke University Press.

Signal, L. 1998. "The Politics of Health Promotion: Insights from Political Theory." *Health Promotion International* 13(3).

Singer, M. 2004. "The Social Origins and Expressions of Illness." *British Medical Journal* 69.

Singer, M., and S. Clair. 2003. "Syndemics and Public Health: Reconceptualizing Disease in Bio-Social Context." *Medical Anthropology Quarterly* 17(4).

Smith, E.R. 2009. "The Canadian Heart Health Strategy and Action Plan." *Canadian Journal of Cardiology* 25(8).

Smith, D.B. 2005a. "Racial and Ethnic Health Disparities and the Unfinished Civil Rights Agenda." *Health Affairs* 24(2).

___. 2005b. "Eliminating Disparities in Treatment and the Struggle to End Segregation. New York: The Commonwealth Fund. <commonwealthfund.org/>.

___. 1998. "Addressing Racial Inequalities in Health Care: Civil Rights Monitoring and Reports Cards." *Journal of Health Politics, Policy and Law* 23(1).

Smith, D.E. 2005. *Institutional Ethnography: A Sociology for People*. Oxford, UK: AltaMira Press.

___. 1987. *The Everyday World as Problematic: A Feminist Sociology*. Toronto: University of Toronto Press.

Smith, J., M. Borchelt, H. Maier and D. Jopp. 2002. "Health and Well-Being in the Young Old and the Oldest Old." *Journal of Social Issues* 58.

Smith, L.T. 1999. *Decolonizing Methodologies, Research and Indigenous Peoples*. London and New York: Zed Books.

Sontag, S. 1972. "The Double Standard of Aging." *Saturday Review of the Society* 1(1).

Soroka, S., R. Johnston and K. Banting. 2007. "Ethnicity, Trust and the Welfare State." In F. Kay and R. Johnston (eds.), *Social Capital, Diversity and the Welfare State*. Vancouver: University of British Columbia Press.

Spence, A. 2008. *Ontario Hunger Report 2008: The Leading Edge of the Storm*. Toronto: Ontario Association of Food Banks.

Spitzer, D.L. In press (2011). "Work, Worries and Weariness: Towards an Embodied and Engendered Migrant Health." In D.L. Spitzer (ed.), *Engendering Migrant Health: Canadian Perspectives*. Toronto: University of Toronto Press.

___. 2009a. "Policy (In)Action: Policy-Making, Health and Migrant Women." In V. Agnew (ed.), *Racialized Immigrant Women in Canada: Essays on Health, Violence and Equity*. Toronto: University of Toronto Press.

___. 2009b. Crossing Cultural and Bodily Boundaries of Migration and Menopause." In L. Hernandez and S. Krajewski (eds.), *Crossing Boundaries*. Cambridge, UK: Cambridge Scholars Publishing.

___. 2007a. *Stress, Migration, Gender and Type 2 Diabetes*. Edmonton: University of Alberta.

___. 2007b. "Immigrant and Refugee Women: Re-Creating Meaning in Transnational Context." *Anthropology in Action* 14(1/2).

___. 2006. "The Impact of Policy on Somali Refugee Women in Canada." *Refuge* 23(2).

___. 2005. "Engendering Health Disparities." *Canadian Journal of Public Health* 96: S2.

___. 2000. "'They Don't Listen to Your Body': Minority Women, Nurses, and Childbirth." In D. Gustafson (ed.), *Care and Consequences: Women and Health Reform*. Halifax: Fernwood Books.

Spitzer, D.L., and S. Torres. 2008. "Gendered Barriers to Settlement and Integration for Live-In Caregivers: A Review of the Literature." Toronto: CERIS Working Paper, No. 71.

Standing Senate Committee on Social Affairs, Science and Technology. 2009. *A Healthy, Productive Canada: A Determinant of Health Approach*. Ottawa: Canadian Senate.

Stanford Encyclopedia of Philosophy. 2007. "Distributive Justice." *The Stanford Encyclopedia of Philosophy*. <plato.stanford.edu/entries/justice-distributive/>

Statistics Canada. 2009. *Family Violence in Canada: A Statistical Profile*. Ottawa: Canadian Center for Justice Statistics. Statistics Canada Catalogue no. 89-224-X.

___. 2008. *Peoples, 2006 Census*. Ottawa: Statistics Canada. Catalogue no. 97-558-XIE.

___. 2007. *University Tuition*. Ottawa: Statistics Canada.

___. 2006a. "How Healthy Are Canadians? Annual Report, 2005." *Health Reports Supplement*. February 7, 9. Statistics Canada Catalogue no. 82-003-SIE2005000.

___. 2006b. *Measuring Violence Against Women: Statistical Trends*. Ottawa: Statistics Canada. Catalogue no. 85-570-XIE.

___. 2006c. "Low-Income Cutoffs for 2005 and Low-Income for 2004. *The Daily* Thursday, April 6.

___. 2006d. "Toronto, Ontario (Census metropolitan area)." Ottawa: 2006 Census of Population.

___. 2006e. *Aboriginal Peoples in Canada in 2006: Inuit, Métis and First Nations, 2006 Census*. Ottawa: Statistics Canada. Catalogue no. 82-003.

___. 2005a. *Women in Canada: A Gender-Based Statistical Report*. Ottawa: Statistics Canada. Catalogue no. 89-503-XIE.

___. 2005b. "Homicides." *The Daily*. Thursday, October 6. Ottawa: Statistics Canada.

___. 2003. *Canadian Statistics: Visible Minority Population, Census Metropolitan Areas*. <statscan.ca/enlish/Pgdb/demo40e.htm>.

___. 2002. "Health of the Off-Reserve Aboriginal Population, 2000–2001." *The Daily*, Tuesday, August 27. Ottawa: Statistics Canada. Catalogue no. 11-001E.

___. 2001. *Aboriginal Peoples' Survey, Canadian Community Health Survey*. Ottawa: Statistics Canada. Catalogue no. 89-589-XIE2000/2001.

___. 1999. "Psychological Health—Depression." *Health Reports* 11, 3. Ottawa: Statistics Canada. Catalogue no. 82-003.

Stephens, J.C., J.A. Schneider, D.A. Tanguay, J. Choi, T. Acharya, S.E. Stanley et al. 2001. "Haplotype Variation and Linkage Disequilibrium in 313 Human Genes." *Science* 293. <http://www.bcgsc.ca/people/angels/htdocs/MEDG505/2003/papers/Stephens_et_al_2001.pdf>

Sterritt, A. 2007. *Racialization of Poverty: Indigenous Women, the Indian Act and*

Systemic Oppression. Vancouver Status of Women's Racialization of Poverty Project. Vancouver: Vancouver Status of Women.

Stewart M., J. Anderson, E. Mwakarimba, A. Neufeld, L. Simich and D.L. Spitzer. 2008. "Multicultural Meanings of Social Support Among Immigrants and Refugees." *International Migration* 46(3).

Stone, D. 1997. *Policy Paradox: The Art of Political Decision Making* (second ed.). New York: W.W. Norton.

Strothers, H.S., G. Rust, P. Minor, E. Fresh, B. Druss and D. Satcher. 2005. "Disparities in Antidepressant Treatment in Medicaid Elderly Diagnosed with Depression." *Journal of the American Geriatrics Society* 53(3).

Sword, W. 2000. "Influences on the Use of Prenatal Care and Support Services among Women of Low Income." *National Academies of Practice Forum* 2(2).

Takeuchi, D., and D. Williams. 2003. "Race, Ethnicity and Mental Health: Introduction to the Special Issue." *Journal of Health and Social Behaviour* 44.

Tang, H., T. Quertermous, B. Rodriguez, S. Kardia, X. Zhu, A. Brown et al. 2005. "Genetic Structure, Self-identified Race/Ethnicity, and Confounding in Case-control Association Studies." *American Journal of Human Genetics* 76.

Tarlov, A. 1996. "Social Determinants of Health: The Sociobiological Translation." In D. Blane, E. Brunner and R. Wilkinson (eds.), *Health and Social Organization: Towards a Health Policy for the 21st Century*. London UK: Routledge.

Tarusuk, V. 2005. "Household Food Insecurity in Canada." *Topics in Clinical Nutrition* 20(4).

Taylor, T., C. Williams, K. Makambi, C. Mouton, J. Harrell, Y. Cozier et al. 2007. "Racial Discrimination and Breast Cancer Incidence in US Black Women: The Black Women's Health Study." *American Journal of Epidemiology* 166(1).

Teeple, G. 2000. *Globalization and the Decline of Social Reform: Into the Twenty-First Century*. Aurora: Garamond Press.

Tenenbaum, D.J. 2009. "Oil Sands Development: A Risk Worth Taking?" *Environmental Health Perspectives* 117(4).

Thurston, W., L. Meadows, D. Este and A. Eisener. 2006. "The Interplay of Gender, Migration, Socio-Economics, and Health." Edmonton: PMC Working Paper Series WP04-06.

Ticoll, M. 1994. *Violence Against People with Disabilities: A Review of the Literature*. Ottawa: National Clearinghouse on Family Violence, Family Violence Prevention Division, Health Programs and Services Branch, Health Canada.

Timoney, K.P. 2007. *A Study of Water and Sediment Quality as Related to Pubic Health Issues, Fort Chipewyan, Alberta*. Fort Chipewyan: Nunee Health Board Society.

Toebes, B.C. 1999a. *The Right to Health as a Human Right in International Law*. Amsterdam: Intersentia.

Tomas, A. 2005. "A Human Rights Approach to Development: Primer for Development Practitioners." United Nations Development Fund for Women (UNIFEM). <http://hrbaportal.org/?p=3719>

Toronto Charter. 2003. "Strengthening the Social Determinants of Health: The Toronto Charter for a Healthy Canada." <depts.washington.edu/ccph/pdf_files/Toronto%20Charter%20Final.pdf>.

Truong, K.D., and S. Ma. 2006. "A Systematic Review of Relations Between Neighborhoods and Mental Health." *The Journal of Mental Health Policy & Economics* 9(3).

Turcotte, M., and G. Schellenberg. 2007. *A Portrait of Seniors in Canada, 2006.* Ottawa: Statistics Canada. Catalogue no. 89-519-X.

UNDP (United Nations Development Program). 2005. *Human Rights in UNDP: Practice Note.* <undp.org/governance/docs/HRPN_English.pdf>.

UNESCO (United Nations Educational, Scientific and Cultural Organization). 2003. "The Stamford Common Understanding." <unescobkk.org/fileadmin/user_upload/appeal/LLP/HisStamford.pdf>.

UNHR and WHO (United Nations Human Rights and World Health Organization). 2008. *Human Rights, Health and Poverty Reduction Strategies.* Health and Human Rights Publication Series, Issue No. 5. Geneva: United Nations Human Rights, Office of the High Commissioner for Human Rights and World Health Organization.

UNICEF (United Nations International Children's Emergency Fund). 2009. *Canadian Supplement to the State of the World's Children, Aboriginal Children's Health: Leaving no Child Behind.* Toronto: Canadian UNICEF Committee.

___. 2007. *Child Poverty in Perspective: An Overview of Child Well-being in Rich Countries, Innocenti Report Card.* Geneva: UN.

___. 2005. *Child Poverty in Rich Countries.* Florence: UNICEF Innocenti Research Center.

United Nations. 2010. *United Nations Treaty Collection: Current Status of the International Covenant on Economic, Social and Cultural Rights.* <http://treaties.un.org/Home.aspx>.

___. 2007a. *United Nations Declaration on the Rights of Indigenous Peoples.* New York: UN.

___. 2007b. "The Human Rights Impact of Climate Change." Office of the High Commissioner for Human Rights. <un.org/climatechange/pdfs/bali/ohchr-bali07-19.pdf>

___. 2006. *"Convention on the Rights of Persons with Disabilities."* Geneva: UN.

___. 2001. "Strengthening of the United Nations: An Agenda for Further Change." Report of the Secretary-General for the 57th session of the UN. <unpan1.un.org/intradoc/groups/public/documents/un/unpan005675.pdf>.

___. 1997. "Renewing the United Nations: A Programme for Reform." Report of the Secretary-General for the 51st session of the UN. Geneva. <http://www.un.org/millennium/documents/a_51_950_add7.htm>.

___. 1989. *Convention on the Rights of the Child.* November 20. Resolution 44/25. Geneva: UN.

___. 1979. *Convention on the Elimination of All Forms of Discrimination Against Women,* December 18. Resolution 34/80. Geneva: UN.

___. 1966. *International Covenant on Economic, Social, and Cultural Rights.* 21st Session. Resolution 2200A/21. UN Doc. A/6316. Geneva: UN.

___. 1966. *"International Covenant on Civil and Political Rights."* Geneva: UN.

___. 1966. *International Convention on the Elimination of All Forms of Racial Discrimination.* December 21. Resolution 2106. Geneva: UN.

___. 1948. *The United Nations Universal Declaration of Human Rights.* Geneva.

___. 1945. *The United Nations Charter.* Geneva.

United Nations Development Group. 2007. "UN Common Learning Package on Human Rights-Based Approach (HRBA)." <undg.org/index.cfm?P=531>.

United Nations Population Fund. 2010. "The Human Rights-Based Approach." <un-fpa.org/rights/approaches.htm>.

Urquia, M., J. Frank, R. Glazier, R. Moineddin. 2007. *Birth Outcomes by Neighbourhood Income and Recent Immigration in Toronto.* Health Reports, 18(4). Ottawa: Statistics Canada. Catalogue 82-003-XWE.

Utsey, S.O., J.G. Ponterotto, A.L. Reynolds and A.A. Cancelli. 2000. "Racial Discrimination, Coping, Life Satisfaction, and Self-Esteem Among African Americans." *Journal of Counseling and Development* 78(1).

Vallee, B. 2007. *The War on Women: Elly Armor, Jane Hurshman and Criminal Violence in Canadian Homes.* Toronto: Key Porter.

Valverde, M., and A. Pratt. 2002. "From Deserving Victims to 'Masters of Confusion': Redefining Refugees in the 1990s." *Canadian Journal of Sociology* 27(2).

van de Mheen, H., K. Stronks and J. Mackenbach. 1998. "A Lifecourse Perspective on Socioeconomic Inequalities in Health." In M. Bartley, D. Blane and G. Davey Smith (eds.), *The Sociology of Health Inequalities.* Oxford UK: Blackwell Publishers.

VanderPlaat, M. 2007. "Integration Outcomes for Immigrant Women in Canada: A Review of the Literature 2000–2007." Atlantic Metropolis Centre (AMC) Working Paper, Halifax: AMC.

Varcarolis, E.M. 2008. *Foundations of Psychiatric Mental Health Nursing: A Clinical Approach.* Philadelphia: Saunders.

Vásquez, J. 2007. *Mental Health in Latin America and the Caribbean.* Part four of "PAHO and the Reformulation of Mental Health in the Americas." <ops-oms.org/English/DD/PIN/mentalhealth_004.htm>.

Veenstra, G. 2009. "Racialized Identity and Health in Canada: Results from a Nationally Representative Survey." *Social Science & Medicine* 69.

Viruell-Fuentes, E.A. 2007. "Beyond Acculturation: Immigration Discrimination, and Health Research Among Mexicans in the United States." *Social Science and Medicine* 65(7).

Vissandjée, B., M. Desmeules, Z. Cao, D. Abdool and A. Kazanjian. 2004. "Integrating Ethnicity and Immigration as Determinants of Canadian Women's Health." *Women's Health Surveillance Report: Supplementary Chapters.* Ottawa: Canadian Institute for Health Information.

Von Faber, M., A. Bootsma-van der Wiel, E. van Exel, J. Gus?ekloo, A.M. Lagaay, E. van Dongen et al. 2001. "Successful Aging in the Oldest Old: Who can be Characterized as Successfully Aged?" *Archives of Internal Medicine* 161.

Vosko, L. 2006. "Precarious Employment: Towards an Improved Understanding of Labour Market Insecurity." In L. Vasko (ed.), *Precarious Employment: Understanding Labour Market Insecurity in Canada.* Montreal-Kingston: McGill-Queen's University Press.

Wallis, M., and S. Kwok (eds.). 2008. *Daily Struggles.* Toronto: Canadian Scholars Press.

Walsh, C.A., J. Ploeg, L. Lohfield, J. Horne, H. MacMillan and D. Lai. 2007. "Violence Across the Lifespan: Interconnections Among Forms of Abuse as Described by Marginalised Canadian Elders and their Caregivers." *British Journal of Social Work* 37.

Walt, G. 1994. *Health Policy: An Introduction to Process and Power.* London, UK: Zed Books.

Warman, C. 2007. "Ethnic Enclaves and Immigrant Earnings Growth." *Canadian Journal of Economics* 40(2).

Warry, W. 1998. *Unfinished Dreams: Community Healing and the Reality of Aboriginal Self-Government.* Toronto: University of Toronto Press.

Wasylenki, D.A. 2001. "Inner City Health (Commentary)." *Canadian Medical Association Journal* 164(2).

Watts, R.J., and J. Abdul-Adil. 1994. "Psychological Aspects of Oppression and Sociopolitical Development: Building Young Warriors." In R. Newby and T. Manley (eds.), *The Poverty of Inclusion, Innovation and Interventions: The Dilemma of the African-American Underclass.* Rutgers, NJ: Rutgers University Press.

Wells, K., R. Klay, A. Koike and C. Sherbourne. 2001. "Ethnic Disparities in Unment Need for Alcoholism, Drug Abuse, and Mental Health Care." *The American Journal of Psychiatry* 158(12).

Wesley-Esquimaux, C.C., and M. Smolewski. 2004. *Historic Trauma and Aboriginal Healing.* Ottawa: Aboriginal Healing Foundation.

White, Kathryn, Maria Sterniczuk, Gabriel Ramsay and Alison Warner. 2006. "Talking Back to Grownups: Healthy Children, Healthy Communities." A Report on the Social Determinants of Health and Middle Childhood in Canada. United Nations Association of Canada. <http://www.unac.org/hchc/files/Talkingbacksm.pdf>.

White, P. 1998. "Ideologies, Social Exclusion and Spatial Segregation in Paris." In S. Musterd and W. Ostendorf (eds.), *Urban Segregation and the Welfare State: Inequality and Exclusion in Western Cities.* London: Routledge.

WHO (World Health Organization). 2010a. *Accelerating Progress Towards the Health-Related Millennium Development Goals.* Geneva.

___. 2010b. "A Human Rights-Based Approach to Neglected Tropical Diseases." <who.int/neglected_diseases/Human_rights_approach_to_NTD_Eng_ok.pdf>.

___. 2010c. "What Is the "Value-added" of Human Rights in Public Health?" <who.int/hhr/HHRETH_activities.pdf>.

___. 2008a. *Commission on Social Determinants of Health Report. Closing the Gap in a Generation: Health Equity through Action on the Social Determinants of Health.* Geneva: World Health Organization.

___. 2008b. *The World Health Report 2008. Primary Health Care: Now More than Ever.* Geneva: WHO Press.

___. 2007a. "Everybody's Business: Strengthening Health Systems to Improve Health Outcomes. WHO's Framework for Action." Geneva: WHO Press. <who.int/health-systems/strategy/everybodys_business.pdf>.

___. 2007b. "Integrating Mental Health Services into Primary Health Care." Mental Health Policy, Planning and Service Development Information Sheet #3. Geneva: WHO Press. <who.int/mental_health/policy/services/3_MHintoPHC_Infosheet.pdf>.

___. 2007c. *Women's Health and Human Rights: Monitoring the Implementation of CEDAW.* Geneva: WHO Press.

___. 2007d. *International Classification of Diseases.* Geneva: WHO.

___. 2006. *Gender and Women's Mental Health.* Geneva: WHO.

___. 2003. *The Social Determinants of Health: The Solid Facts.* Geneva, Switzerland:.

___. 2002. *25 Questions & Answers on Health & Human Rights.* Health and Human

Rights Publication Series, Issue No. 1. Geneva: WHO Press.

____. 2000a. *Women's Mental Health: An Evidence Based Review*. Geneva: WHO.

____. 2000b. *World Health Report 2000: Health Systems: Improving Performance*. Geneva: WHO Press.

____. 1999. *Geneva Declaration on the Health and Survival of Indigenous Peoples*. Geneva: WHO.

____. 1992. *International Statistical Classification of Diseases and Related Health Problems, Tenth Revision (ICD-10)*. Geneva.

____. 1986. "The Ottawa Charter for Health Promotion." Ottawa: World Health Organization.

____. 1978. *Declaration of Alma-Ata: International Conference on Primary Health Care*. Alma-Ata, USSR. September 6–12.

____. 1946. *The World Health Organization Founding Constitution*. Geneva: WHO Press.

Wilkins, K. 2005. "Predictors of Death in Seniors." *Supplement to Health Reports* 16. Ottawa: Statistics Canada. Catalogue 82-003.

Wilkinson, R. 1996. *Unhealthy Societies: The Affliction of Inequality*. London: Routledge.

Wilkinson, R., and M. Marmot. 2005. "Income Inequality and Population Health: A Review and Explanation of the Wvidence. *Social Science and Medicine* 16: 1768–84.

____. 2003. *Social Determinants of Health: The Solid Facts*. <euro.who.int/document/e81384.pdf>.

Williams, D.R. 1999. "Race, Socioeconomic Status, and Health: The Added Effects of Racism and Discrimination." *Annals of the New York Academy of Sciences* 896.

Williams, D.R., H.M. Gonzales, H. Neighbors, R. Nesse, J.M. Abelson, J. Sweetman et al. 2007. "Prevalence and Distribution of Major Depressive Disorder in African Americans, Caribbean Blacks, and Non-Hispanic Whites: Results from the National Survey of American Life." *Archives of General Psychiatry* 64(3).

Wilson, G. 2000. *Understanding Old Age*. Thousand Oaks, CA: Sage Publications.

Witzig, R. 1996. "The Medicalization of Race: Scientific Legitimization of a Flawed Social Construct." *Annals of Internal Medicine* 125(8).

Wolf, R. 2005. "What Is Public Policy?" <http://ginsler.com/toolbox/>.

Woods, M. 2010. "Cultural Safety and the Socioethical Nurse." *Nursing Ethics* 17(6).

Woodward, K. 2002. "Against Wisdom: The Social Politics of Anger and Aging." *Cultural Critique* 51.

Workman, T. 2009. *If You're in My Way, I'm Walking: The Assault on Working People Since 1970*. Halifax: Fernwood Publishing.

Wray, S. 2003. "Women Growing Older: Agency, Ethnicity, and Culture." *Sociology* 37(3).

Wright, E.O. 2003. "Class Analysis, History and Emancipation." In R.J. Antonio (ed.), *Marx and Modernity: Key Readings and Commentary*. Oxford UK: Blackwell Publishers.

____. 1994. "The Class Analysis of Poverty." In E.O. Wright (ed.), *Interrogating Inequality*. New York: Verso.

Young, I.M. 1990. *Justice and the Politics of Difference*. Princeton: Princeton University Press.

Zahariadis, N. 2003. *Ambiguity and Choice in Public Policy: Political Decision Making in Modern Democracies.* Washington, DC: Georgetown University Press.

Zietsma, D. 2007. *The Canadian Immigrant Labour Market in 2006: First Results from Canada's Labour Force Survey.* Ottawa: Statistics Canada.

___. 2006b. "Immigrant Labour Market Outcomes, Selected Age-Sex Groups." In *The Canadian Immigrant Labour Market in 2006: First Results from Canada's Labour Force Survey.* Ottawa: Statistics Canada. <http://dsp-psd.pwgsc.gc.ca/collection_2007/statcan/71-606-X/71-606-XIE2007001.pdf>.

Zola, E. 1978. "Medicine as an Institution of Social Control." In J. Ehrenreich (ed.), *The Cultural Crisis of Modern Medicine.* New York: Monthly Review Press.

Zuberi, T. 2001. *Thicker than Blood: How Racial Statistics Lie.* Minneapolis: University of Minnesota Press.

Zweig, M. (ed.). 2004. *What's Class Got to Do with It? American Society in the Twenty-First Century.* Ithaca NY: Cornell University Press.

___. 2000. *The Working Class Majority: America's Best Kept Secret.* Ithaca: Cornell University Press.